The National Academy of Sciences' Guidelines and *You*

Enough is known, right now, for us to start improving our chances of avoiding cancer by making some changes in what we eat.

This book describes in detail some steps you can take to make your diet more balanced, more varied, more moderate. The simple steps, the livable diet plan, and the tasty dishes described in this book mean that you can put to work, in your life, the knowledge accumulated by nearly a century of scientific endeavor.

If we follow the Academy's guidelines, with creativity and confidence, every meal we set upon the table can become a special expression of love, for those we care about, and for ourselves.

KRISTIN WHITE is a medical writer who has worked on the staffs of the *Medical Tribune* and *Medical World News*. She is a regular contributor to *American Health*, *Medical Month* and *Your Patient and Cancer*.

DIET AND CANCER

Kristin White

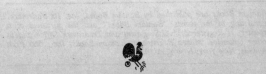

BANTAM BOOKS
TORONTO • NEW YORK • LONDON • SYDNEY • AUCKLAND

DIET AND CANCER
A Bantam Book / July 1984

*This book is not intended to replace
your own physician with whom you should
consult before taking any medication or
considering treatment.*

ISBN 0-553-24246-6

Published simultaneously in the United States and Canada

*Bantam Books are published by Bantam Books, Inc. Its trademark,
consisting of the words "Bantam Books" and the portrayal of a
rooster, is Registered in U.S. Patent and Trademark Office and in
other countries. Marca Registrada. Bantam Books, Inc., 666 Fifth
Avenue, New York, New York 10103.*

PRINTED IN THE UNITED STATES OF AMERICA

H   0 9 8 7 6 5 4 3 2 1

This book is dedicated
with great love
to my remarkable mother,
Cynthia Newman Osterholm.

Contents

Preface

An important finding in cancer research over the past few decades through epidemiological studies demonstrates that the incidence of types of cancer varies widely with geographical location, and is determined predominantly by environmental factors and especially by dietary habits. These findings have raised the exciting possibility of preventing a significant number of cancers through utilization of intelligently planned and properly balanced diets.

Recently, the role of diet in cancer has been subject to a comprehensive review by the Committee on Diet, Nutrition and Cancer of the National Academy of Sciences, U.S.A. These studies have resulted in two reports that present the findings and make specific recommendations for action. While the publications are of immense interest to the cancer specialist, they may not receive the wide readership they deserve from the nonscientific public. Lay readers are too often inhibited in reading reports by scientific bodies.

Now Kristin White has converted these reports into a form that will not inhibit the lay readers. She presents the basic scientific facts on which the recommendations are based in a very readable manner. Most important, she provides a range of specific diets that are in accord with the recommendations of the National Academy of Sciences Committee. Her approach, like that of the committee reports, is both conservative and notably free of faddishness. The information she presents could result in better overall health and a significant reduction in the incidence of cancer among the readers of this book.

Ms. White is to be congratulated on taking practical steps in addressing this important area.

Timothy E. O'Connor, PhD
Associate Institute Director for Scientific Affairs
Roswell Park Memorial Institute, Buffalo, New York

Introduction

As a practicing medical oncologist treating people who have cancer, I have learned to appreciate the suffering, emotional stress, socio-economic changes and the life threatening nature of the disease. Thomas Adams, a 17th century physician stated, "prevention is so much better than healing because it saves the labor of being sick."

Approximately 70% of the causes of cancer may be preventable (32% smoking, 33% diet and 4% alcohol).

The search for a miracle cure, a magic bullet, has not solved the problem. Although the cure rate has improved, cancer still remains our number two killer. The 1983 Data and Figures Report of the American Cancer Society estimated 145,000 of the 440,000 deaths could have been prevented by earlier diagnosis. A larger number of people could also prevent cancer by improvement in life-style, mainly by adhering to current recommendations on diet, smoking, and alcohol.

In 1950, reports in the United States and Britain described the association between smoking and lung cancer. This concept took over 20 years to be accepted, while the deaths from lung cancer have increased from 18,300 (1950) to 117,000 (1983).

In 1982 and 1983, the National Academy of Sciences—The Assembly of Life Sciences—published a report concerning the relationship of diet and cancer, *"Diet, Nutrition, and Cancer."* It is a compilation and summary of all the available scientific evidence of how diet is associated with cancer and proposed recommendations for dietary modifications to reduce the risk of cancer.

Kristin White has simplified the complicated scientific report—explaining and clarifying in a concise, lucid and entertaining fashion, these complex issues. She describes, in an informative, comprehensive way, how our affluent industrialized society's diet—rich in fat, salt and sugar and low in fiber, is dangerous to our health. The rationale and recommendations for dietary change are presented with a "livable diet" consistent with an improved life-style, allowing periodic chances to "cheat." It is of note that these dietary recommendations are the same as the ones for prevention of heart disease, strokes, and diabetes.

We are responsible for our health. We can practice preventitive medicine by adhering to new dietary guidelines as described in this book. Hopefully, we will be able to reduce the risks of cancer in much the same way that cardiologists have reduced the risks of heart disease through improved diet.

Now that we have specific dietary recommendations which may reduce cancer risk, I hope that it will not take as long for the public to begin following them as it did in the case of cigarettes. Kristin White, a respected writer on medicine and a gifted cook, shows us in this concise, authoritative book how urgent and how easy it is for the ordinary person to make these dietary changes now.

Ernest H. Rosenbaum, M.D.
Associate Professor of Medicine,
University of California, San Francisco
Associate Chief of Medicine, Mt. Zion
Hospital, San Francisco, CA.

Acknowledgments

More people helped me to write this book than there is room to thank individually. Those mentioned here represent many others to whom I am equally grateful. My deepest thanks must go to the thousands of investigators who performed the research on which the NAS report is based, and to the indefatigable members of the committee who reviewed, summarized, and evaluated it in their report.

I am grateful for the generous, patient, and often eloquent assistance of the dozens of people I interviewed. The anonymous help of the staff of the U.S. Department of Agriculture's magnificent Nutrition Information Service in preparing the diet plans presented here exemplifies "government service" in the very finest sense.

Four distinguished and very busy scientists, in particular, gave me more of their time and help than I had any right to expect—Dr. Clifford Grobstein, Dr. Walter Mertz, Dr. Selwyn A. Broitman, and Dr. Roswell K. Boutwell. I am beholden to them, and to the many other men and women who have opened my eyes to the intricate beauty of human biology, and the gallant, unperfected art of treating cancer patients. Some are quoted directly, and gratefully, in this book, others made considerable indirect contributions. I want to thank a special few who entered my professional life as expert sources, and evolved into treasured teachers and friends—Dr. Isaac Djerassi, Dr. Kenneth B. McCredie, Dr. Edward Henderson, Dr. Jeane Hester, Dr. Gerald Rosen, Dr. Isaiah J. Fidler, Dr. Margareta Blombäck, Dr. Baruch S. Blumberg, Dr. Robert C. Gallo, Dr. Michael Brennan, Dr. Emil J. Freireich, Dr. Ernest H. Rosenbaum, and Dr. Willie Lijinsky.

I am profoundly grateful to Mrs. Albert D. Lasker, whose

encouragement, good sense, and kindness have meant so much to me, as to so many others.

I always want to thank my editor at Bantam Books, Grace Bechtold, for her overall wisdom and deft editorial hand, and Knox and Kitty Burger for their faith in me.

1

The NAS Report on Diet, Nutrition, and Cancer

Outside the National Academy of Sciences' white marble headquarters, in Washington, D.C., a huge, strangely child-like sculpture of Albert Einstein sits in a leafy corner, contemplating with delight a granite map of the universe. On a steamy June morning in 1982, reporters and television crews made their way past the statue into the academy, to cover an event which could potentially affect the lives of Americans as profoundly as any of Einstein's achievements.

The event was the release of the first of two reports by the academy's National Research Council Committee on Diet, Nutrition, and Cancer—the result of a two-year effort by a panel of thirteen top scientists. Their report summarized and evaluated all the available scientific evidence concerning the way that the foods we eat affect our chances of developing cancer.

In the bare but serviceable auditorium, the committee's chairman, Dr. Clifford Grobstein, presented the report. For the first time in scientific history, he said, scientists understood enough about the relationship between diet and cancer for a responsible, even conservative, committee to recommend how people could improve their chances of avoiding cancer by changing their diet.

In a very real sense, the committee's recommendations, and the news conference that marked their publication, instantly rendered every previous diet plan obsolete.

Their recommendations were these:

Interim Dietary Guidelines

1) *Cut down your fat intake*. The average American gets about forty percent of his or her daily calories from fat,

1

and that's too much. High fat intake is associated with greater incidence of certain common cancers—particularly breast and colon cancer—while lower fat consumption is linked to a lower incidence of these cancers.

The committee says that reducing fat to thirty percent would be "a moderate and practical target," but that's not a hard-and-fast recommendation. The scientific data could justify an even greater reduction, but that might be too difficult for most people.

2) *Eat fruits, vegetables, and whole grains every day.* The more people eat of these foods, the lower the incidence of various types of cancer. The committee emphasized strongly the importance of citrus fruits (which contain vitamin C), dark-green and dark-yellow vegetables (which contain beta-carotene, a source of vitamin A), and the *Cruciferae*—cabbage, broccoli, and related vegetables (which contain chemicals that inhibit carcinogenesis).

But, the committee emphasized, the good reliable information on which this recommendation is founded concerns whole, everyday foods, not individual nutrients. Therefore, they don't advocate nutritional supplements like vitamin or mineral pills. There is too little information about the way that different amounts of specific nutrients affect our risks of cancer. Thus, the committee says they can't recommend high doses of supplemental vitamins and the like—they may not do you any good, and since some of them are toxic at high doses, they might do you actual harm.

3) *Don't eat very much food that's been salt-cured, salt-pickled, or smoked.* This is based on very strong evidence from China, Japan, and Iceland, where people eat large amounts of foods preserved in these ways, and where there is a high incidence of cancers of the stomach and esophagus. Some of these pickling and preserving methods produce high levels of polycyclic aromatic hydrocarbons and N-nitroso compounds—substances which are suspected of causing cancer in humans. (Though the evidence supporting this recommendation is very strong, indeed, it comes from studies of foods that most Americans rarely, if ever, eat, and according to

committee members has much less relevance for the average person in the U.S. than the other recommendations.)

4) *Efforts should continue to keep our food supply free from substances that pose a potential risk of cancer.* These may occur naturally, or they may contaminate food during production, processing, or storage, and it's up to both government, industry, and consumers to maintain food safety.

Sometimes these contaminants are unavoidable, and where this is so, the committee says, permissible levels ought to be established. The food supply should be tested regularly to make sure that those substances don't exceed the allowable amounts. And, adds the committee, carcinogenicity testing of compounds that are added, either directly or indirectly, to foods, should continue.

5) *Possible carcinogens in foods should be identified, and tested to find whether they indeed cause cancer.* Where it's possible and prudent, substances that cause mutations in laboratory tests (but which may not have been identified as cancer-causing) should be removed from food or their concentration reduced as much as possible, the committee says. But, they note, this shouldn't be done if it jeopardizes the nutritional value of foods or introduces new potential hazards into the diet.

6) *Alcohol should be drunk in moderate amounts, if at all.* Particularly when combined with cigarette smoking, excessive drinking has been linked to a higher risk of cancers of the upper gastrointestinal and respiratory tracts.

In addition, the committee urged that the information on the relationship between diet and cancer should be publicized by health and educational agencies, and that the food industry's cooperation should be encouraged in order to implement these dietary guidelines.

"The weight of evidence suggests that what we eat during our lifetime strongly influences the probability of developing certain kinds of cancer," the committee reported. At the same time, it cautioned that it isn't possible now—*and may never be possible*—to lay down dietary rules that can protect everybody against every form of cancer.

Having done, in their view, the best job possible with the evidence available today, the committee pointed out—as if that were necessary!—that science doesn't know everything about the relation between diet and cancer, or even as much as scientists would like to know. More research is going on right now, and new evidence is accumulating almost every day.

The committee, therefore, called their recommendations "Interim Dietary Guidelines," and asked the National Cancer Institute to devise a way for the guidelines to be reviewed and updated at least every five years.

New facts generated by research now under way or about to begin may show new ways that we can modify our diets to reduce our risks of cancer.

Some people might argue that, since the field is new, the information incomplete, and the guidelines themselves not very sensational, the report and recommendations serve no purpose and that we might as well go on doing what we have been doing until something really *definitive* comes out.

But, the committee pointed out in the second report in June, 1983, people *must* make dietary choices every day from a food supply that is rapidly changing. When people want answers, and when those that come from scientific research are at least as good as answers coming from other sources (and probably better), a scientific community that did nothing would "imply that nothing has been learned from several decades of research."

A *lot* has been learned, and although science can't give us all the answers just now, a topflight group of scientists has at least reported on what those decades of research have revealed. The scientists on the NAS committee discharged their responsibilities with what their colleagues consider flying colors. Now it's time for us—the people for whom the guidelines were developed—to assume our own responsibilities.

Even with admittedly incomplete evidence, the message is clear. As Dr. Grobstein, the committee chairman, pointed out at the 1982 news conference, "the evidence is increasingly impressive that what we eat has an effect on the incidence of cancer." While it's frightening to think that our food, our source of strength and pleasure and life itself, can conspire to

4

bring us illness, pain, and death, it's hopeful, too. For we have solid information that we can start *doing things* to reduce that statistical threat that hangs over each one of us.

How the NAS Report Came to Be

The efforts of thousands of research scientists and physicians around the world, working independently but keeping in touch through scientific journals and personal communications, had accumulated a great body of evidence, unorganized and not properly evaluated. Why not assemble an independent panel of experts to simply sit down, sift through all the scholarly articles and reports one by one, weigh the totality of the evidence and derive some sensible guidelines people could use? Why not have this group of scientists identify the gaps in our knowledge, questions which research should focus on in the future, wondered Dr. Sushma Palmer, project director for the National Academy of Sciences.

"This is the kind of job that the academy was set up to do," says Dr. Palmer, a woman of green-eyed good looks and articulate charm who holds a doctor of science degree in biochemistry and nutrition. No longer an active scientist, she now recruits world-class authorities to donate their services to projects for the academy, which serves as a national clearinghouse for scientific information. An authority of almost Olympian prestige on scientific subjects, it's one of the few American institutions whose integrity has never been seriously questioned by anybody.

In June 1980, the National Cancer Institute gave the NAS the mandate to assess where we are today in research on diet's relation to cancer, to "develop a series of recommendations related to dietary components (nutrients and toxic contaminants) and nutritional factors which can be communicated to the public," and, in a second report, to delineate the areas that need more research.

Dr. Palmer rounded up a committee of thirteen eminent men and women, each an acknowledged expert. Most are actively engaged in hands-on research. They brought a wide diversity of scientific expertise.

Some of their specialties are familiar: nutrition, public health, internal medicine, biochemistry, toxicology. Others may sound exotic.

5

Epidemiology, for example, is the mathematical science that looks for the patterns in which disease occurs in large numbers of people, and seeks the meaningful differences between the people who stay healthy and those who get specific diseases.

Molecular genetics is the very special chemistry of the deoxyribonucleic acid molecule (DNA)—the famous "double helix" in every living cell that governs its behavior.

Embryology is the study of how a human being develops, in utero, from fertilized ovum to a full-term baby with all the proper organs—it's also the science of how the cells of the embryo mature and specialize.

The scientists on the committee shared two traits—they are all regarded by their colleagues as first-rate, and all of them came to the committee with a deep sense of the importance of doing the job well. Apart from those common qualities, they differ widely in personality and in their approach to science.

Dr. John Cairns, perhaps the world's leading cell biologist, enticed to Boston from England by the Harvard School of Public Health, is outspoken about what he knows for sure, cautious not to claim too much, particularly when speaking to nonscientists. Dr. Joan Dye Gussow, chairman of Columbia University's Teachers College department of nutrition education, is an energetic consumer advocate. Dr. Thomas Slaga, one of the most respected investigators of carcinogenesis in laboratory animals, is a low-key friendly fellow who looks like a high school football coach. He was working with a new breed of mouse, specially bred for carcinogenesis work, at the Oak Ridge National Laboratory in Tennessee, when the committee was formed; today he's director of cancer research at the University of Texas's new Science Park Research Division.

As an advisor, the NAS brought in Dr. Takashi Sugimura, director of the National Cancer Center Research Institute of Japan, a pioneer in bringing together laboratory research and epidemiology to illuminate the practical ways that diet can affect cancer incidence, and a scientist renowned for inspiring other scientists.

Later in this book, you will meet some of the committee members, vivid individuals, all of them.

To chair the committee, the academy selected Clifford

Grobstein, former dean and vice-chancellor of the University of California's medical school at San Diego.

Now professor of political science and public policy at San Diego, Dr. Grobstein focuses on areas where legislators and policymakers must find common ground with scientists and doctors, places where the problems of technological advances are piling up on our society.

Dr. Grobstein brings a cool practicality to burning issues, recognizing that scientific facts alone can't solve problems and arguing that ordinary citizens and lawmakers alike ought to pay attention where science is able to shed any light. "But," I asked him in an interview after the second report was published, "is it really the government's business to tell people what to eat?"

"I think that just as we expect the government to provide national defense, most people would buy the idea that our government ought to protect the public health," he said. The food supply, which is clearly important to the public health, is no longer a local matter, and thus it's the proper task of the state and federal authorities to see that it's kept safe. "We don't get eggs from Farmer Brown any more—our food is a social product, just as an automobile is. Even so-called natural foods have been processed in some ways—packaged, transported, preserved, refrigerated, marketed. Our food supply is complicated, and it's *national*—even international. We get kiwi fruit from New Zealand these days."

So the government, required by the U.S. Constitution to "protect the general welfare," does indeed have a responsibility to see that people don't unwittingly harm themselves with what they eat, Dr. Grobstein says. "In that sense, the government also has a role in advising people about food."

"But is it really government's job to tell people to reduce the proportion of fat in their diet from forty percent of calories to thirty percent?" I asked.

"That's not a government decree, that's public education, the most minimal form of government involvement," he said, adding that the government has a further responsibility to spread the information around and foster a climate in which consumers can make informed choices—if they want to.

"I'm speaking for myself, not the committee, which didn't

7

address this question," he stressed, "but I certainly wouldn't want the government to change the standards for meat, for example—to say that beef with a fat content above a certain level should not be sold." Instead, he'd rather see the fat content, whatever it might be, specified on the label, so consumers could decide for themselves.

"It would be impossible for a government decree to keep anybody from eating too much or too little of anything," Dr. Grobstein said, then deadpanned: "Fat chance."

Dr. Grobstein's committee were to do no new scientific research themselves—instead, they were to bring their own experience and wisdom to bear on research that had already been performed.

To begin their work, the committee instituted a computer search of the scientific literature which revealed over two thousand scientific articles on the relationship between diet and cancer.

In formal scientific articles and reports, the materials and methods used in the study are described: the strain of rats or mice and the composition of the food or chemical given them; the group of people under scrutiny and pertinent facts about their ages, sex, geographical location, with a careful description of how the information was gathered and analyzed.

Numbers are important—the bigger the better, because, in living things, almost anything is bound to happen once in a while. To make sure that whatever happened in an experiment didn't happen by chance, standard statistical rules are applied. The more animals used in a test, or the greater the number of patients or healthy people surveyed, the more "statistically significant" the results.

These mathematical ground rules are scientists' assurance (and ours) that the evidence that supports conclusions is reliable, not a quirk of luck.

Studies performed by equally careful and qualified investigators, and published in equally prestigious journals, may not arrive at the same conclusions. That doesn't mean that one investigator is "right" and the other "wrong." If each is accurate in reporting what was done in his experiment, and what happened, they're *both* right. A contradiction means that some other factor that wasn't taken into account must be at work.

8

In studies of diet and cancer, there are plenty of contradictions. Living creatures like humans—and mice and even bacteria—are wonderfully complex. Individuals vary in their responses, even when they're genetically identical. Diet, as we shall see, is an extremely intricate factor—really a shifting collection of influences that feed into and affect each other. In this situation, the results of separate studies may not be consistent.

The Work of the Committee

Biology has had no single larger-than-life intellect to grasp all the gorgeous possibilities of living things, as physics had Einstein. The research on diet and cancer alone has been done by several thousand scientists, doctors, mathematicians, and technicians. To organize and draw conclusions from all that evidence would have been beyond any individual—but assigning that task to a committee brought new kinds of problems.

"When we sat down together for the first time, each of us had a point of view, and some of those points of view were initially at odds with others," says Dr. Selwyn A. Broitman, a dean at the Boston University School of Medicine. "We talked, we discussed, we went home and read the articles we were assigned to read, critiqued them, and brought our ideas back to the next meeting and discussed them all over again. We really went at it."

One member's strong conviction that irresponsible, profit-seeking food producers were loading the food supply with carcinogens drew fire from other members at early meetings, who argued that the available evidence didn't support any such sweeping conclusions. Over the months, each member was forced to test preconceived notions against the weight of hard evidence.

As working scientists themselves, the members knew that every scientific study has its limitations. The strongest, most inescapable limitation in biology is the stubborn fact of individual difference. Identical twins may look alike but never lead lives that mirror each other precisely as their physical appearance would suggest; one twin may develop cancer and the other may not.

The same holds true for laboratory rats and mice, inbred so that each animal within a strain is genetically the identical "twin" of the others of the same sex. Some animals develop tumors when given a carcinogen, but others stay healthy, and others undergo changes which aren't malignant, even though all are fed the same food in the same lab and maintained in totally uniform fashion.

A specific dose of an agent—a chemical, a form of radiation, a kind of food—can cause a *range* of effects because individual creatures differ. Some animals respond a little, some a lot, and others not at all. And when the experiment is repeated in a different group of animals, the number that respond in each way may be somewhat different.

In biology, answers are seldom cut-and-dried. The committee, therefore, decided "not to place too much emphasis on the *results*, especially the precise quantitative data . . . from any single study."

Thus, the committee surveyed *all* the evidence, instead of drawing conclusions from separate studies, and set themselves tough standards to judge the total results.

"When they found that different *kinds* of studies, done by different investigators, pointed to the same conclusions, the committee felt that those conclusions had greater merit than those supported by only one kind of experiment," recalls Dr. Palmer.

"And when it came to making recommendations, we agreed that all of us had to be able to live with them," says Dr. Broitman.

"They really confronted issues and debated them," the chairman, Dr. Grobstein, told me with satisfaction. He's not the sort of person who'd have enjoyed presiding over a rubber-stamp process. "There was a fair difference of attitude, and at some of the discussions, it seemed they would never come to an agreement. Then, suddenly, it became obvious to everybody that *this* conclusion was one that all the members would be able to accept.

"All our final recommendations represent compromises," says Dr. Broitman. "Some people think they're too conservative, and individual members of the committee may still feel that certain recommendations don't go far enough."

Though the members are quick to credit the academy's editor, Frances M. Peter, with organizing and writing the report—and reorganizing and rewriting it as their thinking evolved—the final, inch-thick version was truly written by no individual, and by each individual member, sweating over every word.

Their deliberate caution in evaluating the evidence and in deriving recommendations from it led to recommendations that have been compared to "doing what your grandmother used to tell you." They're not sensational. The apparent simplicity adds up to a balanced, varied, moderate diet—with the full weight of modern science behind it.

Where Next?

Once the 1982 report was made public, attention turned to the second part of the NAS committee's task—identifying areas where research should focus in the coming years.

"We solicited comments on the first report from about one hundred people noted for their knowledge of the area," Dr. Grobstein explains. Most of them came to a miniconference in Washington, and discussed with the committee the report and where research should go. "This feedback made the committee more confident about the second report," says Dr. Grobstein. "But I don't think it changed anyone's mind—anyone who's read the first report carefully could have guessed what many of our recommendations were going to be."

The second report, published almost exactly one year after the first, identifies important gaps in our knowledge about diet and cancer and some glaring limitations in our present methods and the tools for investigating them. It points out what else needs to be learned about the different kinds of fats and how the presence or absence of one affects the ability of another to cause cancer. It urges that the research on different types of fiber be studied to see how they affect carcinogenesis, and asks whether fiber has any influence on cancers in parts of the body other than the digestive tract.

"There is a dearth of animal models that are both sensitive and relevant for assessing the influence of diet and nutrition on cancer in humans," they say, and furthermore, the currently used test methods involving animals need to be standardized so that studies performed in different laboratories can be compared. And we've got to have better ways of translating results from animal experiments into meaningful information for human beings, the committee urges. Nobody

11

is really happy with the assumption that if something causes or prevents cancer in a mouse it must necessarily act the same way in a human being.

Today, scientists can't begin to say whether there's a safe dose of a carcinogen in humans, the committee points out, and a method for doing so is sorely needed. We also need a means of studying how initially harmless compounds are transformed within the body to carcinogens and mutagens; at present, knowledge is sketchy, at best.

At the other end of the scale, the committee recognized that, as important as laboratory animals are, not nearly enough is known about the people who will, and will not, get cancer.

A virtually uncharted area is *behavior*, perhaps as vital a factor in the interplay of diet and cancer as any other. What makes people revise their way of eating? When a person leaves home, gets married, loses a job, how does he change his eating habits?

Almost nothing is known about how children learn their eating habits. The committee urges new, long-term studies to determine how food habits become established in early life, since they probably have a crucial bearing on cancer risk later.

We also need to know about what we, as a nation, are really eating, and how it's affected by social factors, a person's life-style, and geographical location. And, the committee urges, this data should be gathered in a way that could be analyzed to show what an individual was eating throughout his life.

As Chapter 9 in this book reveals, vitamins A and C and several minerals apparently have an influence on the development of cancer, but, the committee points out, too little is known about the way these nutrients act in the body. That must be investigated, they urge, and, in addition, people who stand at high risk of developing cancer because of their occupation ought to be monitored over the years to see if the amount of these vitamins and minerals they consume affects their risks of developing cancer. Laboratory studies should be done, the committee says, to find at just what point in the development of cancer these vitamins and minerals intervene to stop carcinogenesis.

The same kinds of studies must be done to discover just

how varying amounts of fats, proteins, and total calories affect the way that certain cancers develop, says the committee. Why is a high intake of fat associated with some types of cancer, and not with others? Can animal studies in the laboratory show us what goes on?

The committee would also like to see research on whether exercise has any impact on cancer risk. No research has been done in the past, perhaps because the profound effects that exercise has on body chemistry have only recently been explored.

Regulatory agencies hold that the only way to discover whether a food additive or contaminant is carcinogenic, observes the committee, is to feed it to laboratory animals. What's carcinogenic in animals is assumed to be carcinogenic in humans. "However, there are no satisfactory methods of establishing, or even estimating, the magnitude of the cancer risk to humans in the amounts they are likely to encounter it," says the committee.

And because such additives are so widely used that just about everyone has been exposed to them, there are no unexposed people to provide a basis for comparison. To be on the safe side, federal regulatory agencies try to keep known carcinogens to the lowest possible levels but, since there are no ways to estimate how great the risk really is, says the committee, "The actual health benefit of this policy cannot be determined."

They offer ten specific recommendations for research on additives, contaminants, on substances known to be carcinogenic in animals, and on mutagens. They urge research to find out how cooking, processing, storage, and the digestive environment affect these compounds, and how much of these compounds are consumed by different groups of people. They urge the development of better assays for carcinogenicity in the test tube, especially using human cells.

An all-out assault to implement the committee's recommendations might very well save the lives of many people who are on their way to developing cancer today but don't know it. A sort of NASA effort on diet and cancer would be a splendid adventure, with unimaginable benefits.

But in the present tight economic situation, that kind of intensive effort isn't going to happen and the committee presented its recommendations in that knowledge. Over the next five or ten years, some research funding will probably be allocated, a little at a time, to answering some of the committee's questions. Perhaps more will follow. The cost of doing long-term studies in human beings or a thorough piece of animal research is immense (for reasons that will be evident in Chapter 6). The committee has set some high, rigorous standards for the way diet and cancer research ought to be done, but quality is not cheap.

But there are other ways of approaching some kinds of research—ways which don't require huge federal investments.

Thousands of American Cancer Society volunteers undertook a massive epidemiological study of dietary and life-style factors in the fall of 1982. They are interviewing one million adult Americans about what they eat, how they cook their food, what medicines they're taking, and a host of other questions whose answers might turn out to affect their cancer risk.

The indefatigable volunteers will do follow-up interviews at two-year intervals, and will keep tabs on which individuals develop cancer and other diseases, and which ones die. New information is bound to emerge and will surely be reflected in the guidelines as they are updated in coming years.

The Purpose of This Book

Despite the limitations of our knowledge and our methods for learning more about the relation between diet and cancer, which are spelled out clearly in the 1983 report, the NAS committee's underlying message is both clear and hopeful.

Enough is known, right now, for us to start improving our chances of avoiding cancer by making some changes in what we eat.

"We don't need to know the precise mechanisms or the reasons why things happen as they do in order to intervene in the development of cancer," says Dr. Ernest L. Wynder, president of the American Health Foundation. "We can act *now*, using the knowledge at hand."

The knowledge at hand is summarized in the two NAS committee reports, both available from the National Academy Press, in Washington, D.C. They are much more comprehensible to the ordinary reader than are most government reports or learned journals, and for doctors, scientists, nutritionists, and students concerned with diet, cancer, or both subjects, these reports will be required reading for years to come.

But these reports aren't likely to attract many nonscientists as readers. They presuppose a certain level of scientific knowledge. And they offer no specific suggestions on how the consumer and the family cook can translate the knowledge gained in the laboratory into action in the kitchen or at the supermarket checkout counter.

This is why I've attempted to present the committee's findings in terms that people with an interest in staying healthy, but without much scientific background, can understand. Of course there is some science in this book—if you know why a thing is so, you can grasp its importance better than if you are simply told, "This is how it is." This book goes into a few of the more significant reasons behind the committee's conclusions—reasons which underscore the importance of starting now, *today*, to make those guidelines work for you.

Much of the latter part of this book describes in detail some steps you can take to make your diet more balanced, more varied, more moderate, as the committee suggests, with special emphasis on the foods science has found to assist our bodies in preventing cancer. There are many practical shortcuts to this better way of eating, a simple diet plan based on patterns developed by the U.S. Department of Agriculture, some sample menus, and some good recipes that use foods available at any supermarket.

This kind of stove-top science was, of course, beyond the scope of the NAS committee, but it shouldn't be beyond yours. The simple steps, the livable diet plan, and the tasty dishes described in this book mean that you can put to work, in your own life, the knowledge accumulated by nearly a century of scientific endeavor.

How much can an improved diet reduce that threat? The committee wouldn't venture even a ball-park estimate, except to say that if Americans all started following the guidelines, we'd see a "noticeable reduction in cancer deaths" by the time twenty years had passed.

So I can't tell you how sure you can be that you'll never get cancer if you follow the principles outlined in this book.

But I'd like to remind you that the committee is *conservative*. They bent over backward to keep their language, and the public's expectations, moderate. My personal judgment is that if this very careful and responsible group of scientists said that the guidelines would lead to a noticeable reduction in cancer, the actual results might very well be better.

Cancer is perhaps the most feared, most destructive disease that threatens human beings. We are all afraid of it. The best way to come to terms with that fear is to take intelligent responsibility for our own lives, and do whatever we can to prevent that disease. It's not only reasonable to follow the NAS committee's advice, it's one way to set our minds at ease. If we follow their guidelines, with creativity and confidence, every meal we set upon the table can become a special expression of love, for those we care about, and for ourselves.

2
What the Dietary Guidelines Can Mean to You

Some of the risks of cancer are built into the human condition and life on earth. Radiation is our constant companion—it comes from the rocks and soil and from cosmic rays. Through evolution, our bodies have acquired protective mechanisms to handle most radiation that we ordinarily encounter, but it's an unavoidable risk factor just the same.

Nor can science eliminate the extra cancer risk that a very few, very unfortunate people have inherited. There are defective genes that can be passed from parents to children, which under certain conditions predispose the offspring to one or another specific type of cancer. These people can be tested periodically to spot the cancer when—and *if*—it develops. For genetically predisposed people live with added risk of cancer, not absolute certainty that it will occur.

If a person has such a predisposition, it's in his or her makeup—and cannot be undone.

There is a brighter side to this dark picture, however. The cancers that kill the most people in Western industrialized countries may be *preventable*.

The NAS committee found a convincing amount of solid, well-documented evidence that whether or not a person develops one or another of these cancers may have something to do with his or her eating habits. Many scientists believe that diet may play a deciding role.

This is good news for everybody. It means that we may have some control over our risks of developing cancer. We don't have to think if ourselves as passive victims, sitting ducks, or prisoners in a hostile environment. There are precautions that we can take, beginning with our diet.

Taken together, the cancers most closely linked to diet account for the great majority of cancer deaths in Western industrialized countries. These are: cancers of the colon and rectum (an estimated 58,100 deaths in the U.S. in 1983), breast cancer (37,500), prostate (24,100), and pancreas (22,300), according to the American Cancer Society.

The major single cancer killer is lung cancer, which caused an estimated 117,000 deaths in the U.S. in 1983, according to the American Cancer Society. Although lung cancer is clearly more related to cigarette smoking than to any other cause, the risks may be modified by changing the diet, even if the person continues to smoke.

The American Diet

Americans have more control over what they eat than any other people in the world. Americans have an unparalleled food-distribution system that brings fresh lettuce from California to Maine in midwinter, and live lobsters to Las Vegas overnight. I never appreciated how staggering our choices are, even in ordinary supermarkets, until I traveled to Eastern Bloc and Third World countries and saw the limited and boring selection of foods millions of shoppers are faced with.

The refrigeration, packaging, and sanitary standards that keep our food from spoiling have spoiled *us*—we reject, automatically, the dirty potato, the imperfect peach. I learned just how high my own standards are while staying at a hotel in the U.S.S.R. on the Black Sea. The Russian guests got all excited one afternoon when word got out from the kitchen that there were fresh apples for dinner that night! These Soviet apples must be pretty special, I assumed.

At dinner, the Russian guests smiled greedily when the fruit was brought on, and they fell to with enthusiasm, while I sat stunned, staring at the tiny, yellow, brown-spotted, sickly looking apple on my plate. It was tasty enough, but not remarkable. Most of the apples harbored worms, but they didn't dampen the Russians' enthusiasm.

I can't imagine fruit of that calibre being served at an American table, or offered for sale at any supermarket.

With our finicky high standards, and with the abundance, freshness, and variety of food offered in our stores, we are surely the best-nourished people in the world—aren't we?

Sad to say, we're only *potentially* well nourished. Good nutrition and terrific health are not the rule in this country. We're *over*nourished in some ways and *under*nourished in others. We take in forty percent of our calories in the form of fat, which is way too high a proportion, and not nearly enough dietary fiber. Why?

It's not because we lack choices or would enjoy a healthier diet less. And surely it's not because we want to pay later with illness, indignity, and early death.

The reasons are complicated. For one thing, people seem to *like* fat. Dr. George V. Mann, associate professor of biochemistry and of medicine at Vanderbilt University, says that when poorer countries become affluent, their consumption of fat goes up. The typical diet in a poor, totally undeveloped country gets ten to twenty percent of its calories from fat; when foreign investment or oil wealth brings prosperity after centuries of crude, monotonous eating, people in Third World countries start eating more and more fatty foods, leveling off when fat calories reach about forty percent of the total.

"We don't know why," says Dr. Mann. "But people all over the world just seem to like fat in their diets if they can afford it."

Another reason for Americans' high consumption of fat is our array of unconscious attitudes toward eating. Ideas like: "Dinner isn't dinner without meat." "Polyunsaturated oils are good for your heart, so they can't be fattening." "Fresh fruit is okay, but I want a *real* dessert."

Through our obedience to these unconscious dogmas we reinforce our own unhealthy eating habits. They lead us into obesity, digestive disorders, and, until a few years ago, a soaring incidence of heart disease. The situation has begun to improve. We've begun to make inroads against heart attacks, stroke, and cardiovascular disease, most experts believe, because we've learned to eat less saturated fat, and because newer breeds of meat-providing animals have less fat than used to be the case. But the reforms we've made have not affected the incidence of cancer. Before the NAS reports were published, nobody was quite sure how our diet affects our cancer risk, or knew what changes ought to be made.

Now, however, we know unquestionably that some dietary

changes could prevent, or at least postpone, cancer in an appreciable number of us. These changes are set forth in the NAS guidelines.

If we are wise and imaginative enough to make these suggested changes in our eating style, we could not only improve our chances of avoiding the kinds of cancer that cause most concern—we could enhance our eating pleasure, too.

For those uninformed, wishful-thinking attitudes lead us into a top-heavy style of eating that is, in its own way, as dull and monotonous as the plain-grain-plus-a-few-vegetables menu in desperately poor countries. There, the choice of food is limited by poverty and politics; in the U.S., many of our meals are limited by affluence.

We can *afford* fat-rich foods and therefore we may feel cheated without the bacon-and-eggs breakfast, the fast-food lunch, the rich evening meal, and the sweet snacks throughout the day. We lose sight of all the other delicious foods. Foods that contain substances that could reduce our risks of cancer.

Can We Change Our Eating Habits?

The committee's recommendations are appropriately conservative and based on well-conducted scientific studies, and even the critics who say that it's premature to tell the public that any diet can reduce cancer risk agree that following these guidelines won't hurt anybody.

But I wondered whether healthy people would want to change the eating habits of a lifetime, to avoid disease that probably wouldn't strike until years later. We are all terribly conservative about our food—Zelda Fitzgerald once remarked that her husband, Scott, not only wanted an egg for breakfast every morning, "he wanted the *same* egg!"

Would people want to make big sacrifices in their eating habits, even for the best of long-range reasons?

I put the question to Dr. Walter Mertz, a thoroughly charming German-born nutrition scientist, and a man who knows how to enjoy life. He is the director of the U.S. Department of Agriculture's human nutrition center in Beltsville, Maryland, and served on the NAS committee.

At the press conference when the report and the guidelines

20

were made public, I asked Dr. Mertz, "Do you really think Americans want to give up eating the things they like, even to avoid cancer?"

"We aren't talking about giving up anything," he said, his voice serious but his eyes smiling. I could tell that Dr. Mertz liked to talk about food, not just as a matter of scientific interest but also because he's something of a gourmet.

"Our number one recommendation is to eat a balanced, varied, moderate diet, made up of lots of different kinds of foods, prepared as interestingly as you can. Sensory appeal—and good nutrition!"

"But the guidelines say that fat shouldn't account for more than thirty percent of a person's calories," I said. "If the average American gets forty percent of his calories from fat, maybe more, then he'll have to cut out a quarter of the fat he's used to eating!"

Dr. Mertz smiled. "All a person needs to cut *out* is the visible fat from meat. It isn't hard to cut *down* on other fat along the way. Our recommendation about fat is a very conservative, mild reduction from a level which we consider excessive."

Like Dr. Mann, he has observed the mysterious way that fat in the diet increases with national prosperity. Old sayings come to mind—living high on the hog, killing the fatted calf, pig rich.

"In my opinion, a diet with forty percent of its calories coming from fat is not a normal diet," Dr. Mertz went on. "The committee is convinced that the guidelines can help people *return* to a normal way of eating. The recommended changes may be profoundly important, but they are not profound changes."

"You mean that we haven't strayed very far off the track, just far enough to add to the incidence of cancer," I suggested. "We're eating a little too much of the bad things, and not quite enough of the good."

"You're putting it a little too strongly. There's nothing in life that's entirely bad or good, and certainly nothing in nutrition. A little of what you consider the 'bad' things won't hurt you, and too much of the good things can cause harm," said Dr. Mertz. So that was what he meant by moderation. It didn't sound too drastic.

There had been a lot of publicity about possible carcinogens in charcoal-broiled foods back in the mid-1970's, so I asked, "Do you mean that a person could eat char-broiled foods sometimes without adding to their risk of cancer?"

"Of course," said Dr. Mertz happily. "I *love* to cook steaks on my backyard grill. I eat them, and enjoy them, and serve them to friends with a good conscience. But not every night, even if I could afford to. I limit it to every weekend or two. But that isn't so bad, because there are so many other good things to eat."

Variety, he had said.

I was beginning to get the idea. I asked him how to cope with an elaborate house party I'd been invited to, where I knew there would be lots of beautifully prepared food and well-chosen wines.

"Enjoy yourself," he said reassuringly. "Eat what you please, have some champagne. You wouldn't indulge yourself like that every day, but on a special occasion it's quite all right, provided you *ordinarily* eat a varied, moderate diet. You can splurge sometimes, if you balance it with light, well-planned meals for a few days before and afterward." This, then, was the balance that went with moderation and variety.

"But even when you're making up for an overindulgence, you should prepare your meals with care. You're compensating, remember, not doing penance. Every meal should be a pleasurable experience. There has to be some *joy* in eating!"

Joy in eating. I couldn't agree more.

Perhaps Dr. Mertz enjoyed his once-in-a-while charcoal-broiled steak *more* because it wasn't an everyday item. Perhaps he was reading my mind, for he said, "The committee doesn't say 'Don't *ever*.' We say 'Don't exaggerate.' "

It seemed, after talking with Dr. Mertz, that the NAS committee's ideas could work for pleasure-lovers like me, as well as for deeply health-conscious people. For me, food has always been an exciting part of life. I find great delight in planning a beautiful meal, shopping for the ingredients, preparing it carefully, and sharing it with people I love. To taste a dish I've never eaten before gives me a thrill of high adventure. (What's in there? Pepper? Ginger, fresh or powdered? Garlic, or onions or shallots? Could I duplicate this dish in my own kitchen?)

With my endless explorations in cookbooks and at restaurants, I was already eating a *varied* diet. By eating lots of different foods, I wouldn't be able to eat too much of any one in particular. *Moderation* would follow inevitably. And with just a little thought, and a couple of new habits, I could probably *balance* my diet in favor of lower cancer risks.

Bonuses from Following the Guidelines

As I thought about it, I realized that the guidelines carry benefits in the short run, too. Anyone concerned about cancer is surely aware of other risks to health. It's nice to know that if you follow the NAS guidelines, you'll improve your overall chances of staying healthy.

Increasing the consumption of vegetables and fruits will necessarily increase the amount of fiber—the collective and rather simplistic term for a group of substances from plants that humans can't digest completely. Fiber acts as a slow, gentle, but very effective laxative. If you have any problems with constipation, the NAS guidelines will correct them.

Fiber can relieve and may prevent hemorrhoids and diverticuli (abnormal pockets and pouches that can develop in the colon and may become infected, sometimes leading to peritonitis and death).

Furthermore, fiber-rich foods make you feel as if you've really *eaten* something. They fill you up, and furthermore, they have to be chewed. This time-consuming, rather noisy activity heightens your awareness of the tastes and textures of the food. That's why eating an apple is more satisfying than quickly swallowing an equivalent amount of apple juice.

Fiber from fruits and from carrots can also, it appears, lower the level of cholesterol in your blood.

The NAS committee's recommendations on fat are similar to the dietary goals issued by Senator George McGovern's Senate Select Committee on Nutrition and Human Needs in 1977. The McGovern committee, too, recommended limiting fat to thirty percent of total calories, suggesting a mixture of one-third saturated fats, one-third polyunsaturated, and one-third monounsaturated.

Perhaps optimistically, the McGovern committee estimated

that if everybody in the U.S. followed their recommendations, there'd be an annual increase in longevity of one full percent annually, a halving of annual deaths from diabetes, a one-quarter drop in deaths from heart disease, and the eighty percent of the citizenry who are overweight would reach their normal weight and stay there. Their recommendations also included less sugar, salt, and alcohol, and more starches, fruits, and vegetables, adding up to an overall reduction in calories.

Since that time, a number of roughly similar diet plans have been put forth by scientific and governmental groups such as the Department of Agriculture, the Department of Health and Human Services, and the American Heart Association. All stress the importance of lowering dietary fat in order to prevent heart disease and stroke.

The dietary guidelines on cancer are not rules for losing weight. They assume you're already within your normal weight range and mean to stay there. I myself fall into that category, according to the charts, but like most people, I'd like to weigh a little less, and it seems that it's easier to gain with each passing year.

Since I began living in accordance with the NAS guidelines, my weight has remained within two or three pounds of where I started. For me, splurges do result in a weight gain, but the added pounds disappear promptly after a few days of low-fat, high-fiber feasting. FEASTING? Yes, indeed. I'll tell you more about that in later chapters.

There is another benefit. I cannot guarantee it, but I think the NAS committee's guidelines may save you some money. This has been my experience, and I live in New York City, where nothing is cheap.

Criticisms of the Guidelines

The NAS recommendations won't hurt you and they will almost certainly bring important general health benefits. But will they help prevent cancer?

Did the committee fulfill its mandate to come up with practical suggestions that could really help the average person avoid the disease or postpone its onset?

There has been some disagreement among scientists. Though

24

Dr. Sushma Palmer, the National Academy of Sciences' project director who oversaw the development of the report, says that the comments the academy has received from the scientific community on the report are ninety percent favorable,'' there has been some dissent.

Some say the report is too conservative.

One critic is Dr. Denis P. Burkitt, the Anglo-Irish surgeon whose years with the peoples of East Africa convinced him that their simple diet of whole grains and vegetables kept them from getting colon cancer. The NAS guidelines contain no specific suggestion that people should increase their fiber; Dr. Burkitt would have liked to see an explicit recommendation.

"It's a simple difference of opinion," he says. "I myself believe that there's enough evidence that everyone should eat more fiber, but the committee decided there wasn't. Since the evidence is increasing almost daily, I think the guidelines will be revised to include such a recommendation before very long."

Nonphysician Nathan Pritikin, director of the Pritikin Longevity Center in Santa Monica, California, says the recommendation on fat is little more than a small step in the right direction. His own rigorous regime limits fat calories to ten percent of the dietary total, the bare minimum a person needs to stay healthy.

"People don't even miss fat after the first week," he says. "I wish the National Academy of Sciences had made better use of this chance to tell the American public that fat is really, really bad for them."

Dr. John Higginson, former chief of the World Health Organization's cancer epidemiology program, agrees with those who describe the NAS recommendations as bland and boring. "They're something like being 'agin' sin," he says. Their conservatisim and obviousness means they will probably cause no harm to anyone who follows them, Dr. Higginson says, but recommendations of any kind are premature.

"Although the report of the National Academy of Sciences has made some quite strong recommendations regarding fat and other nutrients and cancer, the associations are in no way as well established as that between cigarettes and lung cancer," he insists. Though there is a large body of data concerning several types of cancer and the intake of fat in the diet, he says, "a simple causal relationship of these cancers and fat intake cannot be accepted uncritically."

Without downplaying the role of diet, the relationship of dietary components to humans, whether direct or indirect, is, in Dr. Higginson's view, "neither simplistic nor straightforward."

"We aren't really justified in telling large numbers of people to make changes in their life-styles and eating habits," he summed up. "It's premature."

It's unfeasible, argues another critic of the report, Dr. Samuel B. Tove, head of the biochemistry department at North Carolina State University. People simply aren't going to give up meat and dairy products. "Our kids would starve without their Big Macs," he told a meeting of scientists at the University of North Carolina Medical College. But he has deeper misgivings.

"When you're talking about long-term changes in the diet, you must be concerned about *all* the possible effects. You've got to worry about the whole person, and the way those proposed changes may affect his or her chances of developing diseases other than cancer."

One possibility is that, in an effort to avoid dietary fat, people might just stop drinking milk. Going overboard in this way would eliminate the best source of dietary calcium. A long-term calcium deficiency leads to loosened teeth and brittle bones. (The intelligent solution, as you've probably guessed, is to switch to low-fat milk!)

I asked Dr. Mertz about these and other criticisms. Is it, as Dr. Higginson and others suggest, too soon for anybody to make recommendations about diet and cancer?

"A scientist would always like to have more evidence and more figures before going on the record," Dr. Mertz answered. "At the same time, if one holds back and doesn't do anything, the problem continues.

"In considering this philosophical question, which is surely as old as science itself, we thought back to the time, twenty years ago, when the first evidence emerged that suggested that smoking cigarettes led to lung cancer.

"If, at the time, there had been *strong* recommendations,

with the weight of the whole scientific community behind them, many people might have stopped smoking then who are now dying of smoking-related cancers that they could have avoided.

"We're in a similar situation today, with dietary evidence. We don't have enough hard data, certainly not as much as we would like. But there is enough to convince the members of the committee that something should be done—and done *now*.

"So we've issued the guidelines. They are based on the best scientific evidence. If people follow them, beginning today, we honestly believe there'll be a *sizeable reduction in cancer in about twenty years*."

How Effective Will the Guidelines Be?

The committee doesn't offer even a ball-park estimate of "sizeable," even though they knew that an indication of how many cases of cancer the guidelines could prevent would help to "sell" them to the public.

After looking at *all* the evidence, however, the committee concluded that "the data are not sufficient to quantitate the contribution of diet to the overall cancer risk, or to determine the percent reduction in risk that might be achieved by dietary modifications."

Other scientists, looking at their own evidence, have made some educated guesses. We've all heard that as much as ninety percent of all cancer in humans is due to environmental factors, the most obvious of which is diet. Committee member T. Colin Campbell, director of the nutrition cancer program project at Cornell University, told a biennial scientific meeting in Ithaca, New York, that he believed diet to be *the* most important environmental risk factor.

Another estimate is that diet is responsible for thirty to forty percent of cancer in men and sixty percent in women. Two epidemiologists say that dietary modifications would have the greatest effect on the incidence of cancers in the colon and stomach, and a somewhat lesser impact on cancers of the breast, uterus, and lung.

The committee, then, could easily have spiced up their guidelines with some promising numbers. Since the impact of dietary changes wouldn't show up in the cancer incidence statistics for another twenty years, the committee would most likely not be criticized if time had proven their numbers to be wrong. After all, little fudgings with statistics occasionally occur in Washington, D.C.

But not at the National Academy of Sciences, where Einstein is watching.

3

Cancer and Its Beginnings

If you are an average adult, you have about ten trillion cells in your body. To understand how these myriad cells get along together when a person is healthy, and how things go wrong when cancer develops, it's helpful to draw some parallels with the way that citizens interact with each other, politically and economically, within a state or city.

Just as a municipality requires administrators, garbage collectors police officers, messengers, and hundreds of other kinds of workers, the human body needs specialists. Each cell has its own duties to perform; each benefits from the work done by all the others.

Different types of cells not only have different responsibilities, they have different growth characteristics, as well. Some must divide often to replace those that die or are sloughed off. Others divide only under certain circumstances.

In some parts of your body, cell division normally goes on constantly, because certain types of cells are short-lived, and expendable. The cells that line you, inside and out, are used up continually, thrown away, and replaced with fresh cells, because your skin and the inside of your digestive and respiratory tracts are subjected to constant environmental wear and tear. Sunlight, physical irritation, soap and water, kill and damage skin cells. Instead of making them hard and long-lasting, like the shell of a lobster, nature has programmed our skin cells to be temporary, replacing themselves every week or so.

Similarly, we must replace the cells inside us that come in contact with the stresses of our environment as we eat, drink, and breathe. Cells on the inside of the mouth, throat, and

lungs, the esophagus, stomach, and intestines, are all designed to serve briefly and then be thrown away. Their short
life is as carefully planned as the specialized function of the
brain cells which last all your life.

Specialized cells in the bone marrow, when called upon,
provide an army of soldier cells for the immune system.
When you have an infection, each of these bone-marrow
"stem" cells divides into two; the daughter cells divide, and
so on, rapidly. Each successive generation is slightly different
from the previous one; this process, known as *differentiation*,
ends with a host of mature, well-armed white blood cells.
These militant cells, known as lymphocytes, have a single
aim—to seek out, recognize, and destroy the invading virus
or bacteria. That's all they can do. In gaining life-saving
specialization, the mature lymphocyte loses its ability to divide.

In fact, most mature differentiated cells in the body cannot
divide except under specific circumstances, and some do not
divide at all once the body's full adult quota is reached. Brain
cells can't reproduce themselves at all, which is why "brain
damage" from injury or lack of oxygen is permanent. But
other types of cells—skin, muscle, kidney, and so forth—
undergo division within strict controls, to replace dead or
injured cells. Once the lost cells are replaced, cell division
stops. Otherwise, you'd grow yards of new skin when you
cut your finger.

DNA: Rules and Recipes of Life

Your body, then, is a community of specialized, well-
controlled cells. Every community requires a code of law,
and every citizen needs to know the rules that apply to him or
her. Your body's "charter" is codified in a very large molecule called deoxyribonucleic acid, or DNA. Every cell carries
a copy in its nucleus, and when a cell divides in the process
called *mitosis*, each daughter cell inherits a complete copy of
the DNA, this compendium of the rules that make you uniquely
you.

DNA has also been compared to a blueprint, because your
DNA is a plan that includes all your biological qualities—
your sex, your blood type, your straight or curly hair. This
master molecule has also been described as a kind of computer program, because that famous double-helix molecule

consists of thousands of "on" and "off" switches. Just as a keyboard command causes a computer to perform some function, a DNA "switch" instructs the cell to do something, or to stop doing it—to produce a protein, for example, or to begin mitosis so that a new cell can be born.

But since this is a book about food, I'm going to compare DNA to a cookbook. If you think that's a big jump from the legal imagery I used at first, just remember that in old-fashioned cookbooks, recipes were called "rules."

In the DNA molecule, each "on" or "off" switch is called a *gene*, and each gene is in fact a recipe for a protein. When a gene-recipe is copied by an intermediate molecule called ribonucleic acid, and "read" by the cell's chemical-making equipment, the cell prepares a bit of that very specific protein.

The whole process of life is carried on by means of the proteins cooked up in the cells. Special cells in your scalp are continually dishing out a very obvious protein—your hair. Other cellular products are less apparent and more important. For example, "islet" cells in the pancreas produce a protein known as insulin, according to the very precise insulin recipe in your DNA. Released into the bloodstream, insulin controls the way each cell consumes sugar. Insulin is one of the best known of cellular gene products, and because it acts everywhere in the body, its significance is very great, indeed.

But there are hundreds more of these intercellular messenger proteins, each "coded" by an activated gene in a group of specialized cells, secreted into the surrounding fluids, and picked up by other cells. There, the messenger protein interacts with chemicals spelled out in the receiving cells by other genes.

Just as good communication preserves order in a community, clear signals save our multicellular selves from chaos. In our bodies, cells communicate with each other by means of little chemical messages, passed around like cookies or casseroles in a friendly village. It's done with astonishing speed and accuracy.

Each normal cell is a law-abiding citizen, working hard, staying in place, minding its cellular business. A normal cell divides only in obedience to specific chemical messages sent out when the good of the body as a whole demands new cells.

And normal cells stop dividing when they receive other messages telling them, "Enough!"

Cancer develops from cells that escape from the rules. The chemicals that enforce the rules of growth and restraint have, understandably, been the subject of intensive research. Some, such as the "growth factors" that make certain cells undergo mitosis, have been isolated and are beginning to yield some clues about their functions.

But there are many other infinitesimal chemical signals, more mysterious and possibly more important, such as those that pass from cells to neighboring cells which are undergoing division. These signals say, at the right moment, "Hey, it's getting crowded!" Perhaps cancer begins when a dividing cell loses the ability to receive or respond to a complaint from a neighbor.

Cancer-Prone Cells

Whatever specific chemical event constitutes a cell's first step from normality toward malignancy, it's more likely to occur in cells of some types than in others. Ninety percent of all cancer deaths are due to *carcinomas*, the malignancies that arise in the short-lived, quickly replaced, constantly dividing cells of the skin, the linings of the airway, lungs, and digestive tract, the cells that make up breast tissue and some important internal organs. They are derived from the outer tissue of the developing embryo called the *epithelium*.

Cancers in the stolid, long-lived, undividing cells of the brain and nervous system are extremely rare. So are *sarcomas* (cancers of the bone, muscles, and connective tissues) and *leukemias* (cancer of the bone-marrow stem cells that give rise to cells circulating in the blood).

In all, over a hundred forms of cancer are known. They have been diagnosed, catalogued, and carefully observed by physicians and surgeons with increasing precison for a couple of hundred years. The behavior of each type of cancer, the "natural history" of each form of the disease if left untreated, is well known. Although it's impossible to predict just how an individual patient will fare, a doctor who's experienced and well informed can figure the odds with considerable accuracy.

How Cancer Behaves

Scientists know full well why cancer is a disease that nobody should take lightly. These reasons stem from the ability of cancer cells to keep reproducing, while defying the body's frantic signals to stop.

Cancer is *invasive*. Once it's started, a cancer shows no respect whatsoever for neighboring organs and tissues, and pushes through all the natural boundaries. A cancer starting on the inner wall of the colon grows into the intestine's interior space, like mud oozing through a crack in the wall of a tunnel, and it grows outward, erupting into the abdominal cavity, blocking ducts and blood vessels, squeezing vital organs out of position, taking over.

Cancer is also *metastatic*. That is, most cancers spread not so much like crabgrass but like dandelions. Individual cells break off from the original clump, slip into the bloodstream or the lymph, and wander through the body until they come to rest. If one of those wandering metastatic cancer cells happens to settle in a spot conducive to growth, it starts to divide and form a new colony, or *metastasis*.

The whole body may be seeded with mestastases long before the original cancer, known as the *primary*, is big enough to be noticed. Very often, the primary can be wiped out completely with surgery or radiation, but like some super-dandelion spreading its seeds before it blooms, the cancer may already have spread metastases throughout the body. Getting rid of the primary, of course, does not affect the distant colonies that may be too small to be spotted on a scan or X ray. That's why chemotherapy for cancer can make a life-or-death difference. It's the only known way to chase down metastatic cells throughout the whole body.

And cancer is a *killer*. Left untreated, every type of cancer will sooner or later kill every patient who doesn't die first from some other cause. Only early cancers of the skin and of the cervix can be cured with ease. The major cancers are difficult to treat, unless diagnosed very early, when most patients can be treated successfully with surgery alone. Most early cancers cause no pain, and by the time symptoms appear, they are usually so well established that it may be impossible to remove them completely with surgery, or even to determine exactly where in the body the disease has spread.

The people who get these cancers are middle-aged and older—living in what Winston Churchill called "the broad, sunlit uplands" of one's years. For them, cancer treatment means financial and family hardship, time away from work, and, depending on the individual, side effects ranging from unpleasant to dangerous. And for the elderly patient, all-out treatment that offers a chance of cure may be too much for an aged or infirm cancer victim to risk.

Unlike the rare cancers of young people (acute leukemia, testicular cancer, and Hodgkins' disease), which have a cure rate nearing ninety percent, the major cancers are stubborn, and cures are hard-won.

Physicians know the deadly "personality profile" of each kind of cancer. They know that colon cancer's invasive spread disrupts the architecture of the abdominal organs, and that its metastatic takeover of the liver prevents the filtering and purification processes on which life depends. They know that breast cancer metastases follow predictable paths through the armpit's lymph nodes, the bones, the lungs, the brain. They know some cancers of the lymph system shrink readily when treated with almost any anticancer agent, only to counterattack with renewed ferocity; other types may seem to resist treatment, then suddenly disappear weeks or months afterward.

But if treatment doesn't work, or it's too late, the cancer cells keep on dividing, invading, and metastasizing until the patient dies.

How Cancer Begins

Though cancer's outcome for about half of its victims is tragically obvious, how it *begins* is infinitely more complex and only partly understood. This is why the question of how to prevent cancer, by diet or by any other means, is so hard to answer.

It's easy to explain and prevent diseases caused by a single identifiable agent like the smallpox virus or the tuberculosis bacillus. When specific dietary factors are discovered to be associated with particular conditions, people can change their ways and avoid health problems. Pellagra, once a major scourge, virtually disappeared when vitamin A was restored to white flour, and as people have started eating leaner meats and more polyunsaturated fats, heart disease has decreased.

Science has learned much about diet, nutrition, and cancer but knowledge is still incomplete. Without more evidence, the NAS committee was unwilling to go farther than it did in telling the public how to amend their diet.

After all, seventy-five percent of Americans will *not* develop cancer. If people who are healthy today are told to make drastic life-style changes in order to improve chances of avoiding cancer that are already three-to-one in their favor, any recommended changes had better not cause them harm of some other kind. Furthermore, the NAS committee reasoned, people have a right to expect genuine benefit if they alter the dinner-table habits of a lifetime.

Mindful of these responsibilities, the NAS committee chose a course that seemed at first too conservative to some members, and premature to others, but which all eventually accepted. There was enough evidence, in the opinion of the serious, critical-minded NAS panel, for a beginning to be made. As new findings come in, the finer points of the relation between cancer and human nutrition will surely emerge, and as this happens, the NAS dietary guidelines will be refined and made more specific.

In abbreviated form, here are, once again, the dietary guidelines:

1) Reduce the fat in your diet to thirty percent of calories.
2) Eat fruits, vegetables, and whole-grain foods every day, especially citrus fruits, dark-green and deep-yellow vegetables, and cruciferae (cabbage-family vegetables).
3) Limit your consumption of salt-cured, salt-pickled, and smoked foods.
4) If you drink alcohol, do so in moderation.

Initiation

The common killer cancers don't appear to begin as the result of any single cause. Instead, carcinogenesis is a subtle, lengthy *process*.

To embark on that process, a cell has to be prepared.

Geneticist Alfred G. Knudson, director of the Fox Chase Institute for Cancer Research in Philadelphia, has evolved what he calls the "two-hit" theory of carcinogenesis, which, though not definitively proven, is plausible to fit the evidence and illuminate the way dietary factors affect carcinogenesis.

Dr. Knudson theorizes that for cancer to begin, two events must occur in the proper order. The first "hit" is preparatory. It might be a bit of damage to the DNA—a zap of one of a special kind of chemical or a tiny flash of radiation to a critical spot. If the cell's almost-always-effective DNA-repair systems fail, the tiny molecular scar will remain, to be passed on to the cell's progeny during mitosis. Such a DNA change is called a mutation; agents that can cause this type of DNA alteration are called *mutagens*, or change-makers. (In rare cases, the first "hit" may be an inherited DNA defect acquired from the parents, with that DNA anomaly appearing in each cell of the affected person's body, predisposing him to a particular form of cancer.)

We hear a lot about "mutagens" in our food and how dangerous they may be, and many of the chemicals known to cause cancer in laboratory animals are indeed proven saboteurs of DNA. But mutation doesn't *automatically* lead to cancer.

DNA damage is more likely to kill the cell outright or keep it from dividing. Mutation may have no effect at all, for the DNA cookbook molecule is full of blank spaces, apparently carrying no recipes whatsoever.

That first "hit" in carcinogenesis might not even involve DNA. It could conceivably happen to the cell's surface, making it deaf or unresponsive to chemical signals. Whatever its nature, the first hit is not enough to make a cell malignant—it's only the beginning. For this reason, agents that can deliver this first punch are called *initiators*. An initiated cell may live on for the lifetime of the person, and without the second necessary "hit," never become cancerous.

Consider the thousands of Japanese exposed to massive doses of radiation in atomic bomb blasts. Radiation, as we all know, can lead to cancer. But, in contrast to the way most people exposed to influenza virus come down with flu symptoms soon afterward, atomic bomb survivors did not develop cancer right away. There is an increased incidence of some malignancies in these people, but it took years to show up.

No evidence suggests that everyone exposed to those massive doses of radiation will inevitably develop cancer. Other factors must be involved.

Promotion

Carcinogenesis isn't exactly a one-two punch—the second "hit" is more like a series of properly timed nudges.

Our understanding of this phase of carcinogenesis comes largely from experiments on laboratory animals—experiments which had become standard long before the two-hit theory.

The classic way to induce cancer in a mouse is first to rub the skin on the animal's back with one of several well-known chemicals known as—that's right—initiators. Most initiators are mutagens, and are thought to work by causing direct, rapid, irreversible damage to the DNA of the skin cells.

But if the experiment ends with initiation, nothing happens. No cancer, not even any visible changes. To make a cancer develop, the initiation step must be followed with *promotion*, the repeated application of a chemical that modifies or speeds up the normal process of cell division. Many substances make cells proliferate but don't make them malignant. Most promoters used in the laboratory seem to affect chemical reactions on the cell's surface rather than the DNA in the nucleus. Some of these effects may have something to do with that all-important ability of the cell to heed chemical signals from other cells. Cancer researchers would dearly love to know just how promoters confuse cell-surface activities and garble incoming messages.

Researchers would also like to know why timing is so important to carcinogenesis. After applying the initiator, readying the mouse's skin cells, the second promoting process can be postponed for much of the animal's lifetime. When the promoter is finally applied, cancer occurs just as surely as if it had been given right away. Hence the conclusion that once initiated, a cell stays initiated.

The promoter must be given again and again. One big dab of promoter cannot complete carcinogenesis, but when divided into small amounts and administered regularly, the same total dose of promoter leads to cancer. If too much time elapses between applications of the promoter, however, nothing happens, and when allowed to rest long enough between doses, the skin cells reverse their drift toward malignancy.

But the priming effect of the initiator is permanent. An initiated cell can be turned into a cancer cell at any time with the right doses of promoter on the right schedule.

A scenario of this kind is undoubtedly being played out all the time within our bodies. Each of us surely has a number of cells that have been initiated by terrestrial, solar, and cosmic radioactivity, mutagens in our environment and the food we eat. Genetic inheritance adds to the number of initiated cells, accidents waiting to happen, fuses waiting to be lit. The promoters that can complete carcinogenesis are entering our bodies all the time, in what we eat, drink, breathe, smoke, and otherwise ingest.

Furthermore, we ourselves manufacture promoters. Some of the sex hormones—estrogens, for example—can promote cancer. And in the acid environment of our stomachs, nitrogen-rich compounds from important, vitamin-laden foods combine with proteins from others to produce chemicals called *nitrosamines*. Some nitrosamines are cancer promoters. We worry a lot about carcinogens in the world around us, but what about those in the world within?

Is the human body dangerous to our health? So far, it probably sounds that way, but it's only part of the story. The rest is rather wonderful.

How Our Bodies Prevent Cancer

Nature has endowed us with some very clever and effective means for protecting ourselves from the cancer hazards that beset us, inside and out. We know that the protective mechanisms work most of the time because only one person in four ever develops cancer, even though the deck seems to be stacked against us. Now that science is revealing to us just how cleverly our bodies cope, we can start making choices to help those protective processes along, tipping the odds still further in our favor.

First of all, way down at the molecular level, we have enzymes that protect our precious DNA from damage by radiation, mutagens, and cancer-initiating chemicals. These enzymes function like maintenance crews on a highway, traveling up and down the DNA molecule, looking for trouble spots. When they find a section that's damaged, they dig it out of the molecule and patch in a new piece of DNA that conforms to the master plan.

This excision-and-repair process is marvelously efficient in humans, less so in species that don't live as long. Our superior ability to cope with DNA damage is one fact that's often used to bolster arguments that studies performed in animals like rodents, with less sophisticated DNA-repair capabilities, may not be very relevant to humans.

The importance of DNA repair is not something we think about every day. It's dramatized only when the system doesn't work, as in people with a rare, hereditary illness called xeroderma pigmentosum, who can't repair the DNA damage from ordinary sunlight. Unless they avoid the sun completely, they quickly get multiple skin cancers, more extensive and serious than those caused in normal people by years of intense sun exposure. But for most of us, with our ten trillion cells apiece, DNA damage is rarely permanent. The system works, as a rule, and if it fails, we have a backup array of defenses.

We are able to escape injury from many complicated toxins that plants contain to protect themselves from diseases and insects, because our prehistoric ancestors developed strategies to render these toxins harmless. These ingenious biochemical safety systems also function nicely against many of the new molecules that modern civilization has dreamed up.

One safeguard is plain water, which accounts for much of our body weight. Water is a splendid solvent, an electrical conductor which attracts electrically charged substances (such as metallic poisons) and swooshes them through the kidneys and into the urine. Fatty, oily, complicated substances (like most organic chemicals) are neutral in charge, and not soluble in water. Many of them are toxic and some are carcinogenic, so we have detoxifying enzyme systems which step-by-step chop these big molecules into smaller pieces, adding electrical charges, and rendering them water soluble.

The Amazing Antioxidants

Another important line of defense neutralizes potentially harmful chemicals before they have a chance to pose a threat. Some everyday nutrients strengthen these defenses.

Chemical reactions depend on differences in the electric

charges of one atom and another, between a molecule and its environment. Little packages of negatively charged electrical energy known as *electrons* are the medium of exchange for chemical transactions. Like all other chemical processes, the biochemical events that add up to life depend on the transfer of electrons—in the same way that a community's economic life depends on money changing hands. The chemical transaction is called *oxidation* or *reduction*, depending on the point of view. (If that sounds complicated, just remember that the same transaction can be called either a purchase or a sale, depending on the side of the counter you're on.)

A compound which is giving up electrons is being *oxidized*, one which is collecting electrons is being *reduced*.

Some years ago, Drs. James and Elizabeth Miller of the McArdle Laboratory for Cancer Research at the University of Wisconsin discovered that many compounds known to be carcinogens share an interesting quality. They are electron-spendthrifts, readily oxidized.

The Millers studied known carcinogens and found that when these molecules enter the body and react with fluids and tissues, they start giving away their electrons like a lottery winner on a spending spree, ending up in debt! Newly electron-poor, these oxidized molecules are now ready to acquire electrons. They've become *electrophilic*, or electron-loving, ready to bind indiscriminately to any molecule able to share some of its electrons.

Electrophilic compounds are dangerous troublemakers; they can steal small pieces called methyl groups right out of the DNA, they can bind with RNA, the messenger molecule within the cell. They can combine with proteins to form new, harmful compounds, or act as promoters on cells that have already been initiated.

A lot of oxidation goes on inside the digestive tract, as food is broken down into usable components, sometimes creating carcinogens from foods that started out safe and wholesome. In the acid environment of the stomach, in the presence of other foods and digestive juices, we can create formidable cancer promoters.

You have a great many electrophilic molecules in your body at this very moment, and more are being created all the time. Some come from molecules that came from outside, most result from oxidation reactions necessary to life.

Happily, there are compounds which prevent oxidation from getting out of hand. They're called *antioxidants*—we produce some ourselves, and we get others in food.

Dr. Bruce N. Ames of the University of California, Berkeley, has found that uric acid, present in near-saturation levels in human blood, is an extremely potent antioxidant. Once thought to be just a nasty waste product, uric acid, says Dr. Ames, keeps electrophilic substances from accumulating. "I think it's what keeps us from going rancid all the time," he says.

Many ordinary foods contain antioxidants, a fact which the NAS committee dwelled on at length in their report, and which is reflected in the guidelines.

The vitamin C in citrus fruits, tomatoes, and other foods prevents nitrosamines from forming in the stomach, because it's a very good natural antioxidant. So, too, is vitamin E, available in a wide variety of everyday foods, especially whole grains. The trace element selenium is a key ingredient in an important enzyme which acts as an antioxidant. (More about all these powerful protectors in the chapter on micronutrients.)

In addition, there is a common food additive called BHA, which keeps food from "spoiling." Spoilage is just a homely term for oxidation, and as we note in the chapter on food additives, if BHA can retard oxidation in food, perhaps it can do the same for you.

And there are other protective substances, some identified, others tantalizingly obscure. We know what foods they're in, but not what these compounds are. Others, possibly the most important, aren't even suspected. They do their job so well that we aren't even aware of them.

The combination of cancer-protective substances in our foods, and our own marvelous defense systems means that for most of our lifetimes, most of us do not develop cancer.

I discussed this once with Dr. Roswell K. Boutwell, of the McArdle Laboratory at the University of Wisconsin. "You know," he mused, "we keep finding so darn many chemicals that cause cancer in our laboratory animals. Not just new chemicals that industry has dreamed up, but substances that have been around as long as humans have been.

"If all these things caused cancer in *us* as efficiently as

41

they do in rats and mice, we'd all get cancer soon after birth.''

"Well, why don't we?" I asked.

"I think we must have better defenses against cancer than these animals do—and most of the time, our bodies are doing a lot of things *right*."

Dr. Boutwell, whose work, dating from the 1940's to the present, is cited frequently in the NAS report, and is regarded as a dean of carcinogenesis studies. Lately he and his team have been concerned with the many specific steps in cancer promotion, not just with testing individual compounds to see if they cause cancer.

"The more we know about the details of carcinogenesis, the more likely we are to find places where we can do something to interrupt it.

"I sometimes think that instead of spending all this time and money to find what chemicals cause cancer, we should pay a lot more attention to the ways we've found through evolution to avoid it," says Dr. Boutwell.

4

The Diet-Cancer Connection

Two basic facts give us a clarifying perspective on how diet affects a person's risks of cancer. First, cancer is not a uniform disease. Malignancies behave similarly, but they originate in many different organs of the body.

Second, the human diet, throughout the world, is by no means uniform, either. People in different countries have strikingly different diets, and there are further differences among the eating habits of people in different social, religious, and economic groups.

The rationale underlying research into the diet-cancer connection comes from the simple observation that the predominating types of cancer vary from one country to another, and that the differences tend to correspond to national differences in what people eat.

Throughout the Western industrialized world with few exceptions, colon, breast, and prostate cancers are major killers. However, colon cancer is quite uncommon in the Third World. Breast cancer, for most of this century, was rare among Japanese women; prostate cancer occurs less frequently in Japan than anywhere else in the world.

At this point, many people may begin to wonder what relevance the diet and the cancer incidence in other countries could have to those of us who live in the United States and eat a typical American diet. Why not study *ourselves*?

The reason is that in science, particularly in matters of biology and health, insight comes from *comparison*. Taking different groups of people, comparing the kinds of cancer they develop, and noting the differences in their diets enables

43

us to perceive patterns, trails of evidence leading to possible explanations whose validity can be tested.

If we are interested in whatever impact that diet might have on breast, colon, and prostate cancer, the next step is to find the major differences in the American and Japanese diets. One big contrast is glaring—Americans consume about forty percent of their calories in the form of fat, while the Japanese eat only fat to account for about fifteen to twenty percent of their calories. To check whether high fat intake could have something to do with high incidence of these cancers, we look at the fat consumption and incidence of breast and prostate cancer in other countries. And we find that throughout the Western industrialized world, the fat in the diet and the rates of breast, colon, and prostate cancer in the people are consistently higher than in other countries.

Comparisons help make sense of what would otherwise be an overwhelming mass of statistics and measurements. Throughout the NAS report, the committee refers to studies done in far-flung countries where both the daily diet and the national patterns of cancer differ from those in the U.S., and the international flavor of the evidence is reflected in this book. Don't assume that, because studies were performed among people who live differently from Americans and whose risks of cancer are not the same as ours, the evidence gained by these studies has no relevance to your own life. On the contrary, the differences make comparison possible, and mean that studies performed half a world away could help you avoid developing cancer.

Genes or Diet?

It has been suggested that people in different countries develop different types of cancer because their genetic heritages are not the same.

Could it be that, like skin color and hair texture, genes for predispositions and resistances to particular cancer exist, and are passed on to enough people within a country to give it a particular pattern of cancer?

We now know that *diet is much more a factor in determining cancer risk than is heredity*, thanks to some large-scale "experiments" unwittingly performed over the past couple of hundred years.

44

These experiments have been done whenever a large group of people has moved en masse to another country. In time, a "migrant group" begins to abandon its old-country ways, adopting the dietary habits of the new home. More than a generation may pass before the impact of the dietary changes appears in the progeny of the immigrants.

"In general," says the NAS committee, "the incidence of cancer in migrant groups is similar to that of the country of origin, or intermediate between that of the country of origin and the host country. After one or more generations, it becomes the same as those of the host country."

If genetic inheritance determined whether or not a person developed one of these cancers, then migrants would retain the same patterns of cancer as the people in the country they left, wherever they moved in the world. And the children of migrants would inherit these patterns. This isn't what happens.

These trends have been studied in specific details for stomach, colon, and breast cancer among Japanese who moved to Hawaii and the U.S. West Coast; Eastern Europeans who migrated to the U.S. and Canada; Icelanders who relocated to Manitoba; and Southern Europeans who went to Australia. The lessons to be learned are consistent.

The change in cancer incidence is slowest for breast cancer, not showing up for a full generation or perhaps two. Migrant women and their daughters develop the disease at about the same rate as women who stayed at home. This may mean that whatever determines breast-cancer risk happens *early* in a woman's life—an important point for parents to remember when planning the family meals.

With colon cancer, and to some extent stomach cancer, the shift in risk is faster. There may be more or fewer cases of this disease among the migrants themselves, than among people back in the homeland, indicating that whatever contributes to the development of colon cancer could be modified in *adult* life. By adopting a new style of eating, for example.

The eating habits that linger among immigrant groups may result in different kinds of cancer incidence between these people and their descendants and others of different background, and nowhere in the world is this clearer than in the U.S.

Ethnic groups usually have some well-defined patterns of eating and drinking which may persist through several generations without much change even though they've adopted most American dietary habits. The Irish, for example, are traditionally drinkers of beer and whiskey rather than wine. Northern Europeans eat little rice and far fewer vegetables than do Orientals. The culinary heritage may not be carried on intact from generation to generation, but the details that are retained may have a crucial effect. A seemingly simple difference, like using oil rather than butter for cooking, may affect cancer incidence.

Where the facts have been analyzed, the NAS committee concluded, "The operation of environmental factors, as distinct from those of genetic origin," made the difference.

Cancer and the Environment

What about other environmental factors apart from diet—the industrial pollutant toxic wastes, and pesticides? Aren't they causing a cancer epidemic?

If we leave out lung cancer—it's the leading killer cancer in the U.S., but most of it is attributable to one factor and you know what that is—and skin cancer (often unreported since it's so easily cured), we find that cancer incidence changed very little for the three or four decades leading up to 1971.

Of course there are more *cases*. There are more people and the population is older. Cancer incidence is greater in older people, but statistical age adjustment allows for that.

If the environment were as horrendously carcinogenic as we have often feared, the factors that have been introduced in recent decades would make it easier for cancer to begin. Cancer would increase among *young* people: becoming less a disease of aging and more significantly a disease of middle age and young adulthood.

But the figures for the past four decades indicate that if anything, the reverse is happening. While very old men seem to be getting more cancer than they used to, middle-aged men have a slightly lower incidence, and among people under forty, especially women, cancer incidence is *falling*! That would not be the case if our world were in fact more riddled with carcinogens than was the world of our grandparents.

We should note, however, that in 1973, the National Cancer Institute Surveillance, Epidemiology, and End Results (SEER) Program instituted new statistical and data-collection methods. After 1973, the data appear to show a slight rise in cancer incidence.

That might mean that the effects of a mucked-up environment are at long last showing up as additional cases of cancer.

Or it could mean the cancer-watching system has been doing a better job since the changes in information-gathering methods, the way a powerful new vacuum cleaner collects more dirt than a feeble old clunker. The NAS committee leans toward the second view, saying that the streamlined methods used since 1973 make it difficult to compare new figures with those before 1973.

As new data accumulate, over the next few years, the question will be resolved and we'll know whether the post-1973 rise is real or a statistical blip.

Any change that may have occurred is *small*.

Though our human carelessness and ingenuity have devised some remarkable new ways to harm ourselves, we haven't as yet caught up with nature's clever coping mechanisms. The very same DNA-repair and carcinogen-blocking systems that guarded our ancestors against natural radiation, viruses, plant toxins, and heaven-knows-what prehistoric biochemical hazards continue to protect us from new dangers.

"We've inherited the defenses that early man invented, and our bodies use them to protect us from the newer compounds," says Dr. Roswell K. Boutwell of the University of Wisconsin. "Don't forget that from the time life on earth began, volcanoes and fires were emitting polycyclic aromatic hydrocarbons. Sitting around in those caves, our ancestors must have gotten almost as much stuff in their lungs as cigarette smokers do today. Life evolved in the presence of molds and toxins and through evolution humans developed defenses. Those that didn't tended to die off."

That's not to say that environmental irresponsibility is either morally defensible or harmless to your health. We *ought* to clean up after ourselves. But the possibility that man-made chemicals will give cancer to everybody is not at the top of the list of reasons to keep our planet tidy.

Or, as Dr. Frederick Becker, director of research at Houston's M.D. Anderson Hospital once told me, "If we're surrounded by a sea of carcinogens, we've learned how to swim pretty well."

Cancer, Diet, and You

I know people who, when they hear some famous person had died from cancer, say, "Well, with pesticides and nuclear power and pollution, it's a wonder we *all* don't have cancer!"

Sometimes I try to explain that cancer has much more to do with factors we have some immediate control over, like smoking and diet, than with carcinogens in the world at large, but they don't want to hear it. They blow smoke in my face.

It almost seems some prefer to believe that cancer is inflicted on us by vague outside forces. They seem to feel most comfortable as *victims*—passive, powerless, and doomed. Perhaps this helpless attitude releases them from responsibility for their own lives and health. If they know in their hearts that the communists, or big businesses, or some other band of high-tech terrorists have set up the environment so that cancer is inevitable, then it doesn't matter how much they smoke. Or what they eat. They can't win, so why bother?

I don't agree. I think life is precious, and good health is perhaps even more precious. Both are worth a bit of effort.

If I should develop cancer, I want to know I've done all I can to avoid it.

To move away from lazy fatalism and into life-affirming, positive action, we must know what we're really eating. What are the substances that make up our food, and in a healthy human body, what purpose does each one serve? And, most important for our purposes, what effect does each one have to raise or lower the risks of cancer?

The answers aren't complete or definitive, but enough is known to work out an eating style that skirts the major risks and lines up the most potent allies on your side.

In the next two chapters, we'll look at the two major tools that scientists use to gather this information. Understanding a bit about epidemiology and laboratory animal experiments will not only help show how the NAS guidelines were evolved and why we should pay attention. It will also enable you to make up your own mind about the value and validity of new research data as it's made public in the future.

5
Tools of the Trade: Epidemiology

In searching for the causes of any disease, investigators employ two main types of studies. *Epidemiology* is the study of the distribution of diseases among groups of people and the factors that determine which people develop or avoid them. *Experimental* methods attempt to study the disease in the laboratory, in artificial systems designed to eliminate confusing influences. In studying diet, nutrition, and cancer, the systems most often used generally involve small, inexpensive, genetically pure strains of rats and mice, but sometimes other creatures are used—monkeys, rabbits, and bacteria, for example. Occasionally, studies are done in human volunteers.

Neither epidemiology nor experimental science is refined enough to reveal the small, subtle differences in the behavior of either people or molecules that may have big impact on our chances of getting cancer. A number of fine, sober scientists therefore argue that the NAS guidelines are premature—we just don't know enough, they say.

But in the committee's view, the very crudity of today's methods makes the conclusions more credible. We had better pay attention to them, the committee implies, because they're *obvious*.

Epidemiology: Patterns of Cancer in People

For our purposes, epidemiology is the attempt to match people's eating habits with their risks of developing one kind of cancer or another. It's *not* fortune-telling and can't predict whether an individual will or will not get cancer.

The great strength of epidemiology is that it focuses on *people*, eating real foods in human-size portions. What they eat is metabolized according to the rules of human biochemistry, which isn't quite the same as that of rats, mice, monkeys, or bacteria.

Furthermore, some people, typically, will ingest more of a particular food than others do, so it's often possible to assess dose response—the relative effects of a substance at different levels of exposure. The essence of dietary studies is to determine whether there's such a thing as a safe dose of a compound that could be harmful at higher doses, or a minimum level necessary to normal health of a substance supposed to be good for people.

Because epidemiologists focus on people, their conclusions aren't extrapolated from facts about other species—a built-in logical weakness in experiments on laboratory animals. Remember the uproar when saccharin was found, in a Canadian study, to cause bladder cancer in mice? Nobody wanted to believe that what was true for mice was necessarily so in man.

The NAS committee considers two types of epidemiological studies most reliable—the *prospective cohort* study and the *case-control* study.

A cohort is a group of people whom you keep track of (with tests, interviews, and meticulous recordkeeping)—over years. A prospective cohort study begins with meticulous baseline measurements of the relevant characteristics of each person, such as medical history, the levels of specific compounds in the blood, and a complete set of blood-cell counts. These tests may be repeated periodically, when the members of the cohort are interviewed again to determine what types of diseases they may have developed and how their living habits may have changed.

A dietary case-control study starts, as it were, at the other end. The investigators start with a group of people who have already developed a particular type of cancer. These, of course, are the *cases*. For each patient, they find a *control*—a healthy person, identical to the patient in age, sex, race, socioeconomic status, and as many other relevant ways as possible.

Each person in the case-control study is interviewed about his or her food intake over the years. Such interviews are conducted by trained workers, asking an extremely broad range of questions, in precisely the same way, of both the patient and the control. Ideally, if the controls are well matched, the only dietary differences that emerge are those relevant to the biggest difference between the two people—the fact that one has cancer and the other doesn't. Some years ago, sociologist Saxon Graham at Roswell Park Memorial Institute in Buffalo, New York, found in a case-control study of colon cancer patients that their eating habits differed from matched controls in only one significant way—the controls frequently ate raw, sliced tomatoes, and the colon-cancer patients did not.

But in humans, the length of time between the first exposure to a cancer-causing agent is usually quite long—twenty years or so. This is called the *latency period*. Even in laboratory animals, promotion takes months of repeated, low-dose exposure; with our superior DNA-repair systems, detoxifying enzymes, antioxidizing methods, and our larger bodies and longer lives, the development of cancer is a long-drawn-out business, and cancer epidemiology takes decades.

Case-control studies are complicated by the latency period. People don't really remember their eating and drinking habits of twenty years ago. (What did you have for lunch last Wednesday? How often did you eat french fries between the ages of fifteen and twenty-five?) The memories of a person under the stress of being a cancer patient may be even more unreliable. Epidemiology has other built-in drawbacks, too. It's rare that epidemiology can turn up answers so clear-cut as the cause-and-effect relationship between cigarette smoking and lung cancer. Most epidemiological answers simply indicate that a higher or lower risk of cancer goes along with a specific activity or type of exposure. It's a long way from figuring the odds to predicting the future.

This is important to remember whenever we hear that scientists have discovered a higher-than-expected incidence of cancer among people who share a particular eating habit, or who work in the same industry, or live in the same place.

We are spoiled, of course, by the statistical wizardry that gives us election-night results only moments after the polls have closed. If computers can tell us, on the basis of a few sample precincts, who won and who lost long before the actual votes have been counted, we reason, they ought to be able to tell us whether a particular chemical in our food causes cancer or keeps us from getting the disease.

But election analysis, complex though it is, is infinitely simpler than epidemiology. Interviewers outside polling places can easily ask people which candidate they've voted for, and since elections are conducted in the same way, year after year, analytical techniques improve each time.

Epidemiologists are faced with a much more difficult set of problems when they set out to look at the relationship between cancer and diet. You could say that, by choosing a Republican or a Democrat, a particular voter cast the key ballot in an election, but it's impossible to say whether, by choosing a hot dog over a grapefruit at a particular meal, a person developed cancer as a result.

Even if we know a specific food to be a surefire cause of cancer—and nobody knows of *any* food that is—its effect on a group of people who ate it regularly would be hard to assess. Some people would eat more of that hypothetically cancer-causing item than others. The foods eaten along with it might, as we'll see, make a big difference. Some people in the group could have an inborn resistance or sensitivity to the food's ability to cause cancer.

The complexity is multiplied when epidemiologists look at groups of people to see whether particular foods protect against cancer. This is why responsible epidemiologists won't say that they've found something *causes* cancer—even though television and newspaper reporters often rephrase epidemiological findings to make them sound more definite and more exciting. The epidemiologists themselves talk about *associations*, not causes.

When they find that people who develop a particular cancer have something in common which is lacking among the people who don't have cancer, epidemiologists say there's an *association* between that factor and the risk of that cancer. A high incidence of colon cancer is associated with a high-fat diet—that's called a *positive* association. A high intake of dietary fiber is associated with a low incidence of colon cancer—a *negative* association.

Association, of course, may be no more than coincidence—some things really are a matter of luck. A basic chore of the epidemiologist is to determine mathematically how probable it is that seemingly associated factors could have occurred together by chance. Against this background, the strength of the association, positive or negative, is silhouetted. If there's a big difference between what you'd expect from coincidence and what you observe in an epidemiological study, then that association is potentially very important.

And where there isn't an appreciable difference between chance and the results of a study, epidemiologists say the difference isn't "statistically significant."

People make fun of that term because it sounds prissy and nit-picking, but it helps separate solid knowledge from fascinating flukes and misleading coincidences. For example, some people are worried about cancer because many of their relatives have died from it. Let's say that of ten of your deceased relatives, three have died from colon cancer, one of breast cancer, one of prostate cancer, two of lung cancer, two of heart attacks, and one in an automobile accident.

"Does cancer run in my family?" you wonder. Seven deaths by cancer out of ten seems like a very high incidence, when you know that the national average is one in four.

An epidemiologist looking at this family would ask first of all if those two lung-cancer patients were smokers, and if they were, he'd point out that this form of cancer is *rare* among people who don't smoke and never have. He'd ask the age of the man who died of prostate cancer, noting that the incidence is very high among older men and that any man of seventy has a seventy percent chance of having prostate cancer. Colon cancer, the commonest non-smoking-related cancer in the U.S. (124,000 new cases estimated in 1983), and breast cancer (114,900 estimated new cases in 1983) are also so common that even when several cases occur in one family, the statistical likelihood is so great to begin with that the surviving people in this family are not, in fact, at any elevated risk. All those cancer deaths resulted from malignancies so very common that the seemingly high prevalence of cancer in the family is really just a sad statistical coincidence.

In other words, before drawing conclusions from the cancer incidence in any group of people, large or small, you must do some statistical homework.

Social, economic, and political homework are important, too, to avoid incorrect but seemingly logical conclusions. To illustrate the kinds of traps epidemiologists can fall into, Richard Peto, an eminent epidemiologist from the University of Oxford, likes to show, with unassailable Monty Python logic, that telephones cause cancer.

Peto—one of those fast-track young scientists who haven't paused to acquire the supposedly indispensible Ph.D.—has collaborated with Sir Richard Doll, director of the Imperial Cancer Research Fund's unit at Oxford, for years. Their studies, including the epidemiological quests that led to the cigarette–lung-cancer connection, are regarded highly because they focus rigorously on the point at issue and don't assume that the obvious answer is necessarily the right one.

"If you look at the statistics, you see more cases of cancer in industrialized countries than in less developed countries," says Peto in his best Oxford-gadfly style.

"Now look at the statistics on telephones. Highly developed countries have many more telephones than does the Third World. A strong positive association exists between the number of telephones in a country and the incidence of cancer. Therefore, telephones cause cancer!"

The association masks other factors, Peto explains. Highly industrialized countries have not only telephones but other high-technology factors: good sanitation and widespread vaccination; lots of doctors and nurses; elaborate systems of recordkeeping.

Poorer countries have poor sanitation and lack preventive-health measures. Many people die early from diseases other than cancer. They have few hospitals and health professionals, so that many people with cancer may go undiagnosed. Undeveloped countries can't afford carefully kept health records, so the people who do develop cancer and who are properly diagnosed may not all be recorded in the medical statistics.

"High-technology countries—with lots of telephones—have an apparently high incidence of cancer, and low-technology countries—with few telephones—have an artificially low statistical incidence of cancer," explains Peto.

In other words, epidemiological studies may answer questions you aren't asking. Mindful of this possibility, the NAS committee decided to be cautious about a chemical precursor of vitamin A called beta-carotene.

On the strength of eighteen out of twenty epidemiological

studies of people in various countries, it looks as if eating foods containing beta-carotene is associated with below-average risks of some cancers. Does beta-carotene, or the vitamin A into which the body converts it, have some cancer-thwarting effect? Maybe.

Should we all race down to the health-food store and stock up on beta-carotene pills? The committee doesn't think so. Those studies don't really *show* that beta-carotene lessens cancer risks in people who eat lots of food containing this substance. It's found in carrots, as you'd infer from the name, and in dark-green leafy vegetables, and all of them contain lots of other chemicals, vitamins, minerals, amino acids, and so on. The foods that contain beta-carotene and have some cancer-preventing effects could very well contain some other real but as-yet-undefined chemical that actually does the anticancer work, the committee reasoned.

Or perhaps a highter-than-average intake of beta-carotene really means that the person is eating less of other foods that increase cancer risk. Maybe. We'll take a closer look at the existing knowledge about beta-carotene in Chapter 10.

Epidemiological studies have a way of yielding answers that are more ''maybe'' than yes-or-no, and in science, maybe isn't an answer. It's a slippery little rascal that must be grabbed and squeezed until the real answer pops out. In epidemiology, maybe means that the same question has to be asked again, in a more refined way.

It's evident that, as a tool for determining the relation between diet and cancer, epidemiology is far from perfect. Or, as Dr. Selwyn A. Broitman, a member of the NAS committee from Boston University Medical School, puts it, ''Trying to find out anything about diet and cancer with even the best epidemiological methods is like trying to operate on the lens of the eye with a pickax.''

At the same time, argues Oxford's Richard Peto, epidemiology is a potentially powerful tool. ''All we need to do is ask the right questions in the right way in order to discover practicable ways of preventing cancer.''

But epidemiology can't make these discoveries on its own. Information from other scientific disciplines is needed, and therefore we turn to the animals.

6
Tools of the Trade: Laboratory Studies

Laboratory Animal Studies

A study conducted in the laboratory is a little like testing a model of an airplane in a wind tunnel—a small-scale reenactment of the real thing. It's cheaper, faster, and provides a new perspective. Details can be adjusted, one by one. By isolating the effects that each minuscule change can have, scientists accumulate specific bits of information.

An animal study starts with at least a hundred rats or mice, specially bred so they're genetically identical. They're divided into groups—the number of groups depends on the particular questions you're asking—with the same number of males and females in each. The groups are fed, watered, and otherwise handled in exactly the same way, except that in one, the *test group*, the animals get the dose of the drug, nutrient, or carcinogen you are studying, or the diet that lacks the factor you want to know more about, or the repeated dabs of tumor-promoting agent on the same place on the skin of the back.

The other animals are the *controls*. No animal study is kosher without controls to provide the basis for comparison, the contrast that highlights the findings and gives them definition.

"The more controls there are, the better the experiment and the information obtained," says Dr. Roswell K. Boutwell, the University of Wisconsin carcinogenesis pioneer. A subtle and sophisticated scientist, he has the directness and simplicity of a Wisconsin farm boy—a very, very smart farm boy.

"If there are exceptions to something I'm investigating, I

56

want to be darn sure that *I'm* the one who finds them out. I don't want some other investigator to publish an article six months later saying Boutwell is all wet!''

Carcinogen Testing in Animals

"In planning any experiment, you need both positive and negative controls,'' Dr. Boutwell explains. "You need to know how often the animals you're working with get cancer when nothing special is done to them. So you have negative controls, treated the same way as the test animals, which don't receive the compound you are investigating in the experiment.

"And to establish the upper range, to show what happens to these animals when they're exposed to something *really* carcinogenic, you have positive controls, which get a really potent, well-studied, standard laboratory carcinogen.

"The animals that get the test compound will probably develop a number of tumors somewhere in between. But when the number is close to either the positive or negative controls, that's really something!''

The more complicated an experiment, the more control groups it needs. If your carcinogen must be dissolved in a solvent such as water or acetone, then a group of negative controls must be dosed with that solvent, exactly the same as the animals receiving the carcinogen.

Dividing the test animals into high-dose and low-dose groups adds another crucial dimension to the study, showing how strong any carcinogenic effect may be.

Common sense says that if a given amount of something has a particular effect, twice as much of it ought to do twice as much. Hitting a baseball twice as hard should send it twice as far.

But because different compounds are broken down and metabolized in the body in different ways, doubling the dose of some dramatically increases the effect, and doubling the dose of others makes no noticeable difference.

"For every compound, there's an ineffective dose, and an effective dose range, and a level above which the effect is overwhelming and toxic,'' says Dr. Boutwell. "This is probably true of carcinogens. Unless an experiment includes dose-response data, it just isn't sound science.''

If a substance is only feebly carcinogenic, small amounts may produce no more than the background number of tumors in the test animals. In this way, a potentially dangerous material could get a clean bill of health. Ridiculously high doses of the compound must be used, even if humans encounter it only in small amounts.

Even with high doses of a carcinogenic compound, not every single animal who receives the test compound will develop cancer. If a carcinogen can induce cancer in one percent of the animals, administering it to fifty males and fifty females won't show you in a statistically satisfactory fashion whether the compound really causes cancer, since one percent of untreated control animals might well develop cancer spontaneously.

In all, testing a single compound for carcinogenicity involves about three years and well over half a million dollars.

To get results reliable enough to make a carcinogenesis test worthwhile, a scientist must use an army of animals, the actual number depending on the number of different control groups needed. There must be a clean, safe place to house them, laboratory staff to tend them properly and administer the test compound and the positive and negative control materials accurately and on schedule, and to keep meticulous records. After the test is completed, statisticians must analyze the data, a job that may take months.

It will yield an answer something like this: "Under the conditions of this particular study, the compound was [or was not] found to promote tumors in this strain of laboratory animals." Not very satisfying to ordinary people who want to know whether it's all right to drink diet soda.

Responsible scientists hesitate to judge food or chemical either safe or dangerous for humans on the strength of just one experiment in animals; on the other hand, two studies of the same suspected carcinogen can't really be compared unless all the factors are identical—the strain of animals used, the food they're fed, and so forth.

Often it seems to happen that a week after the newspapers have said that a substance has been found to be carcinogenic, they report another study showing it's harmless. The differences could well be due to what seemed to be minor matters when each scientist was setting up his study.

Cocarcinogens

Testing suspected carcinogens individually—auditioning each one as a soloist—can't tell us everything we need to know about them. Evaluated one by one, they may prove to be virtually harmless. Many scientists suspect, however, that the big cancer threat comes from the buildup of *small* doses of wishy-washy initiators and promoters over the years, not from a powerful carcinogen a person may encounter once in a lifetime.

Weak initiators and promoters probably perform in ensemble as *cocarcinogens*. Cocarcinogenicity goes beyond the way the compound acts—and into a host of interactions with thousands of others. Scientists have scarcely begun to come to grips with cocarcinogenicity, which is simplicity itself compared to the effects of *diet* on carcinogenesis. Some of those other, inevitable, chemicals present in test animals, and in humans, are likely to be initiators and promoters themselves. And some may even have both initiating and promoting abilities. The best known of these is smoke from cigarettes.

The birth of a human cancer is an elaborate drama, not a clear cause-and-effect event, as we have seen. It happens within a living body, with all kinds of other chemicals present, not just the initiator or promoter being tested.

Testing Foods in Animals

In the laboratory tests, the suspected carcinogens are generally pure substances, and it isn't hard to know how much is being administered. But in investigating the effect of a food on cancer incidence in laboratory animals, new difficulties arise.

Laboratory animals are too small to eat much of anything, and like humans, animals thrive best on a diet that provides just enough of all the right nutrients. When drastic changes are introduced the whole intricate system can be thrown out of whack.

A regime artificially high in some nutrients is likely to cause health problems unrelated to cancer. When a scientist tries to compensate, by adding or removing other nutrients, he tilts the biochemical balance still further. Other scientists in the field will be quick to ask whether his results are due to the extra vitamin, mineral, or other dietary component—or to some indirect effect that the experimental design did not take into account.

I asked Dr. Boutwell how he'd set up an experiment to study whether a specific food, like brussels sprouts, had any effect on carcinogenesis.

"To study this, we might use animals whose cancer incidence is in the normal range, and induce tumors with a chemical initiator and a promoter. We'd use a feeding tube if we are particularly interested in studying a gastrointestinal cancer, or apply them to the skin on the back, which makes the process easier to watch, step by step."

"How can an experiment on the skin tell you what would be going on *inside* the animal?" I wanted to know.

"It makes sense because the cells of the skin are epithelial cells, and the cells that line the gastrointestinal tract and the cells of breast tissue are all epithelial, too. Studying carcinogenesis in the skin gives us a pretty good idea of what may be taking place in other epithelial tissues, where most human cancers start."

After deciding on the appropriate setup, or "animal model," the rest of the experiment has to be planned. "We'd give some of the animals brussels sprouts instead of part of their regular diet, and see how many tumors developed," said Dr. Boutwell.

"And the more controls the better?"

"Right," replied Dr. Boutwell. One group of controls would get the initiator plus the promoter, receiving a normal diet.

"And I suppose you'd need another group of normal animals receiving a normal diet, to establish what their normal incidence of cancers would be," I said. It looked as if a scientist was obligated to include a group of controls wherever it would make an experiment more complicated.

"The problem is that diet studies involve more than one variable," he explained. "The agent that causes cancer is one variable. The diet that's perhaps going to change the incidence of tumors is another. You need more controls than you would if you're just trying to see whether something causes cancer or not."

And, as with humans, life-style factors affect laboratory animals, who experience none of the stresses and dangers of

60

living in the wild. Cages are roomy and kept scrupulously clean, temperature and humidity are comfortable; food and water arrive fresh daily.

The cushy life of animals in control groups leads to problems. "They aren't picky eaters. They eat what's set before them, and they get fat! I've seen rats in control groups that look like they're half the size of a volleyball," says Dr. Boutwell. That may affect the results.

"We have lots of evidence that obesity predisposes to cancer, both in animals and humans. So when the control animals become obese, they may develop more tumors than they would normally. This can throw the results of feeding studies way off balance."

In the past, diets fed to animals in different carcinogenicity and nutrition experiments were seldom comparable. They ranged from garden-variety commercial chow like the kind you feed to the family gerbils, to fancy artificial diets in which a cocktail of amino acids in specific amounts replaces the usual crude protein. The differences in diet may have affected the results of hundreds of experiments. In 1977, scientists finally began to adopt a practice that would help make experiments done by different investigators in different laboratories somewhat easier to compare—since that time everybody has been feeding the same basic diet to experimental animals.

The NAS committee believes that this step will eliminate some of the apples-and-oranges confusion about studies done since 1977. However, the reform won't make studies done before the uniform diets were adopted any easier to sort out.

Why Not Use "Human Guinea Pigs?"

All animal studies have one great drawback—they aren't conducted on human beings.

Man is much better suited biologically to life on this planet than almost any other species. Life expectancy in the United States is over seventy years, and there are scientists who say that if conditions are right, any human body will function well for over a century.

By contrast, rats and mice live about two years. Their protective mechanisms against aging, cancer, and other diseases don't have to work as well as ours. There may be more

61

similarities between humans and rodents than between either species and alligators, worms, or jellyfish, but that doesn't mean that we're the same as other mammals in every respect.

Some of those differences may be extremely important. One reason why the legendary experimental animal, the guinea pig, is rarely used in experiments like those we've been describing is that guinea pigs lack a number of enzyme systems that humans (and rats and mice) possess. Guinea pigs don't adequately mirror what takes place in humans, nor, to some extent, do rats and mice.

On the other hand, human beings don't make very good guinea pigs.

Experimentation on humans is rigorously limited by laws and by the constraints that scientists impose on themselves. This is borne out by the hue and cry that's raised in the scientific community whenever a physician tries a new treatment on patients without having laid careful laboratory groundwork, and without showing that the risks to the patient are likely to be outweighed by the potential benefits.

The vast majority of scientists, particularly those in Western countries, shudder when the possibility of "experimenting on patients" is raised, unless experiments are sanctioned by ethics committees in the hospital, and, at least in the U.S., unless the patient is told what the physician proposes to do and gives his informed consent.

Ethical and safety considerations are even stronger when it comes to testing drugs or diets on people who are healthy to begin with. An all-brussels-sprouts diet couldn't be tested, even in people who volunteered enthusiastically, unless it had first been shown in animals that it wouldn't cause damage. "First of all, do no harm," is the first stricture of the Hippocratic oath, and while I know few physicians who can recite the rest of it, that's the phrase they all can quote verbatim.

But there are overriding practical reasons for not experimenting with humans.

We're genetically diverse, we're too big, we live too long, and we *are* picky eaters. For the *long-term bioassay* studies that the NAS committee gave most weight to, the type discussed in this chapter, human beings would make terrible experimental animals.

Once in a while, however, dietary studies have been done among healthy volunteers. These studies are ethical and useful only when the nutrient being tested is regarded as quite harmless, and when the volunteers conform conscientiously to the requirements of the study. Human studies, therefore, have often been conducted in populations such as prisoners, mental patients, and other residents of institutions where it's relatively easy to control what's eaten and to reduce opportunities to cheat.

But some scientists question whether the sedentary, regimented lives of confined subjects are enough like those of ordinary people, living freely, for the results to be completely convincing. Most other human volunteers come from among the students at the institution where the research is being done. Again, it's not universally accepted that these young, healthy, active people, with the very special stresses of the academic life, really approximate the typical adult American.

Testing in Bacteria

At the other end of the spectrum of tools now used for evaluating components in our diet, there's the Ames test, developed in 1975 by University of California–Berkeley biochemist Bruce N. Ames—the same Dr. Ames who's delving into the role of uric acid as an antioxidant.

The Ames test is a cheap and speedy way to see if a compound can alter DNA and cause mutations—possibly harmful and perhaps potentially carcinogenic. Instead of using animals or humans, the Ames test employs a special strain of bacteria—*Salmonella typhimurum*—and requires only days, not months or years. The test is simple: the compound under scrutiny is mixed with the enzymes it would encounter in a person's liver, to change it into the form it would have in the body, and the enzyme-treated compound is introduced to the bacteria. If the bacteria develop mutations, the compound has the ability to interact with DNA, and is said to be a mutagen.

That's all the Ames test really tells us. It doesn't say whether a mutagen is strong or weak, not tell us for certain that it "causes cancer." Clearly, a mutagen, acting at exactly the right spot on the long DNA molecule, might serve as the first "hit" in the two-step carcinogenesis scenario.

Around eighty percent of the compounds known to be

carcinogenic in laboratory animals are also mutagenic in the Ames test. However, some potent carcinogens, notably chlorinated hydrocarbons, aren't mutagenic to the bacteria, and some compounds that cause mutations in the Ames test aren't carcinogenic to animals. Scientists by no means agree whether mutagenicity to bacteria reflects a compound's threat to humans, for bacterial DNA is not exactly like that of mammals.

Some eminent scientists believe that the concordance between mutagenicity in the Ames test and carcinogenicity in animal systems is plain coincidence.

The NAS committee noted: "It is generally agreed, but not without considerable controversy, that there is a high degree of correlation between the mutagenicity of compounds in the Salmonella . . . assay and their carcinogenicity in laboratory animals." To cancer researchers, therefore, a compound that causes mutations in bacteria is one that merits closer study.

If an ingredient or contaminant in your favorite food is found to be "mutagenic," as measured by the Ames test, it doesn't mean you'll die of cancer if you ever swallow another mouthful. It does make sense, of course, not to overindulge in foods that contain mutagens—charcoal-broiled meat and fish, for example, certain wild mushrooms, and bracken fern (a wild green rarely eaten in most of the U.S.).

How Epidemiology and Lab Science Work Together

In 1976, I attended a meeting at the Cold Spring Harbor Laboratory near New York City. Dr. Takashi Sugimura showed some appetizing photographs of fish, grilled Japanese-style over an open fire, and announced that the charred spots were full of mutagens formed as molecules rearranged themselves at the high cooking temperatures. In the Salmonella test, they caused mutations.

"But do they cause cancer?" he was asked again and again by reporters.

"We won't know whether these mutagens are also carcinogens until we test them in animals," Dr. Sugimura kept repeating patiently.

I asked Dr. Willie Lijinsky about those mutagens in the fish. Dr. Lijinsky, chief of carcinogenesis research at the Frederick Cancer Research Center in Maryland, is one of the world's top experts on carcinogens.

"Do you think those mutagens of Dr. Sugimura's are carcinogens?" I asked.

"I think some of them probably are," he said.

"How do you know?"

"Oh, you can tell just by looking at the molecular structure," he said, whipping out one of those Bic pens that scientists always seem to have about them, and drawing some diagrams on the back of the conference program. The basic architecture of the mutagens in the grilled fish resembled that of some well-known carcinogens.

Circumstantial evidence, but good enough to convict, as they used to say around the courthouse, or so I thought.

"Now, these carcinogens in the fish . . ." I began.

"We don't *know* that they are carcinogens."

"But you said . . ."

"I said I thought some of these mutagens probably are carcinogenic," he said stubbornly, as I felt a good story slipping away.

"But if that's your considered opinion . . ."

"It's my *guess*. I think it's a good guess. But we can't say for sure unless we test these chemicals in animals. A mutagen may be a carcinogen, but a good many of them are not."

"What should I say in my story?" I begged desperately.

"Write your story in a couple of years. You don't have a story now," he said, and after thinking about it awhile, I realized he was right.

The story was a bit riper in the fall of 1982, when Dr. Sugimura—the same Japanese scientist who served as an advisor to the academy committee—presented new findings to the Thirteenth International Cancer Congress meeting in Seattle, Washington.

His findings illustrate the way that different kinds of science take cues from each other. Eventually the different routes converge.

In Dr. Sugimura's lab, a group of animals has been living luxuriously on a diet of which a full ten percent is grilled sardines. The study isn't complete but the animals are developing hyperplasia in their stomach tissues. Hyperplasia, an abnormal and excessive growth of cells, is a condition that can lead to cancer. The control animals fed on regular chow are developing no hyperplasia. Meanwhile, epidemiologists from the National Cancer Institute of Japan are getting some important evidence from northern areas along the Sea of Japan, where studies show people eat a great deal of grilled fish (as well as grilled meats, fried foods, and salt-pickled vegetables), and where statistics show the stomach-cancer incidence is among the highest in the world.

Salmonella tests for mutagenicity show that the hearty grilled diet of the north is very high in mutagens, compared to that of the south, where blander foods prevail and food is seldom grilled.

Though definitive conclusions can't yet be drawn to link mutagens in grilled foods with high risks of stomach cancer, it's an area from which answers should be coming in the next few years. And it's a good example of how different sciences contribute to our understanding of diet and cancer.

No single type of study can tell you, for sure, that a food or a compound either causes or prevents cancer.

No type of study can yield answers quickly. The Ames test provides helpful leads, but offers only a saving in time, not a fast, definitive answer. The answers come slowly, from animal studies that take years, and from epidemiological studies that may take even longer.

How, then, was the NAS committee able to come up with its interim dietary guidelines?

They did it by finding the areas where evidence gathered in independent ways supported the same conclusions. They reviewed *all* the available evidence on diet and cancer, and refrained from deciding anything on the strength of just one study—or on just one type of research.

In formulating their dietary guidelines, the committee looked for areas where there was lots of evidence, all in agreement, and where epidemiological and laboratory data concurred.

Those are strict standards. Since, as we've seen, both epidemiology and laboratory methods are imperfect, it's hardly surprising that the committee's recommendations are few in number and general in language. The committee were all too aware of the limitations of the evidence they had to work with.

Nevertheless, among all that evidence there was some that met the criteria, and the conclusions it pointed to were inescapable. These are the few rosy ripe apples in the bushel of green ones, and they are probably the most urgent conclusions likely to be drawn about diet, nutrition, and cancer.

Though other guidelines will be forthcoming, those issued by the NAS committee are the ones we'd better take most seriously.

Now let's examine for ourselves the scientific evidence from both laboratory and epidemiological studies that shows how the various foods we eat can affect our chances of getting cancer.

7
Fats: The Greasy Villains

"Avoid fried foods. They angry up the blood," enjoined baseball immortal Satchel Paige—long before the American Heart Association, the margarine manufacturers, or anyone else started telling us to start eating lean.

Though people love their fatty foods, and though words like "buttery," "creamy," and "rich" convey the idea of luxury and "the good life," not very many of us nowadays believe that fat is *good* for us.

Maybe that's why so much more research has been done on the relation of fat to cancer than on any other dietary factor. Unlike many areas of diet-and-cancer research, this one *has* some unequivocal answers for us, although some provocative questions remain.

The NAS committee concluded in its report, "of all the dietary components it studied, the combined epidemiological and experimental evidence is most suggestive for a causal relationship between fat intake and the occurrence of cancer. Both epidemiological studies and experiments in animals provide convincing evidence that increasing the intake of total fat increases the incidence of cancer at certain sites, particularly the breast and colon and, conversely, that the risk is lower with lower intakes of fat. . . . In general, the evidence from epidemiological and laboratory studies is consistent."

Satchel Paige, no doubt, could have put it more eloquently, but for a committee of cautious, conservative scientists, that's not bad at all.

One reason they didn't come out even more strongly about the dangers of excessive fat is that, particularly in Western diets, fat is tied to the consumption of other nutrients. We rarely eat pure fat; we eat it in foods—meat, cheese, butter, and sauces. These contain other, more complicated substances, and it can't be said with absolute certainty that fat intake *alone* increases the risks of colon, breast, and other cancers.

But the evidence is quite convincing that if you have already quit smoking cigarettes, the next big favor you can do for yourself is to adopt a leaner cuisine.

A number of international studies show that, more than anything else in the diet, fat consumption is higher where colon and breast cancer rates are high, low where these cancers are uncommon. Whether they examined marketing statistics for fatty foods, or individual consumption from personal interviews in case-control studies, the committee found breast and colon cancers associated with a high intake of fat.

There is also a strong link between fat and cancer of the prostate, though the data are more limited. A striking increase in mortality from prostate cancer has taken place in Japan since 1950, simultaneously with dramatic changes in the Japanese diet, from traditional low-fat, fish-rice-vegetable fare to fattier Westernized diet complete with franchised fast food. In addition, there's some association between dietary fat and cancers of the testes, the uterus, and the ovary.

Fat and Colon Cancer

The evidence concerning fat and colon cancer is perhaps most interesting, however, because of the number of people affected, and because the risk can be lowered in *two simple ways*.

If we set aside the tobacco-caused malignancies, cancers of the colon and rectum kill more Americans than any other form of the disease. It's depressingly common throughout the industrialized world, and though curable if diagnosed early enough, most colon-cancer patients reach their physicians after the disease has metastasized to the liver, making cure unlikely.

Study after study shows that countries with high fat consumption have a high incidence of colon cancer. In countries where colon cancer is common, you also find high incidences of cancers of the breast, uterus, ovary, and prostate. With monotonous regularity, around the world, these cancers are common where people eat large amounts of fat, and low where fat is a small part of the diet.

In Bombay, the poor, vegetarian Hindus have substantially less colon, rectal, and breast cancers than the richer, meat-eating Parsi population who, in turn, have less of these cancers than do people in the West.

The Seventh-Day Adventists, who abstain from smoking and drinking, and about half of whom follow a diet permitting milk and eggs but no meat, have a much lower risk of dying from colon or rectal cancer than the average American. They have a lower risk of breast cancer, but the difference is less pronounced. The committee speculates that since many Seventh-Day Adventists have converted to the religion as adults, their risk of breast cancer may have been determined early in life. The new dietary ways may have been adopted too late to change their breast-cancer risk, but early enough to reduce their chances of colon cancer.

The traditional Japanese diet derives fifteen to twenty percent of its calories from fat. Over the past twenty-five years, Japan's consumption of fat has been creeping upward and, recently, the Japanese incidence of breast cancer has begun to climb.

Japanese women who have migrated to the United States, trading their traditional diet for American fare, retain their low risk of breast cancer. Second- and third-generation Japanese-American women, however, acquire the same degree of risk as other American women.

So it appears that at any time of life, a high-fat diet increases the risks of colon cancer, while too much fat in girlhood adds specifically to a woman's risk of breast cancer.

Fat and Fiber

Now for the good news about fat. The effects of fat that increase cancer risk can apparently be reduced considerably by *fiber*.

"You can really get away with eating some fat, if you defend yourself by eating enough fiber," says Dr. Denis P. Burkitt, the internationally renowned advocate of high-fiber diet. "The emphasis in scientific circles is shifting away from the idea of fat as a carcinogen toward fiber as a protector."

A study of men in Scandinavia, whose hearty appetites

lead to a high consumption of cheese, sausages, creamy sauces, and other rich foods, showed that while the sophisticated Danes had a high risk of colorectal cancer, the earthy Finns' risk was low. The big difference in their diets was that the city-dwelling Danes liked white bread, while the Finns ate lots of coarse peasant rye bread and other high-fiber, whole-grain foods.

We'll discuss fiber in greater detail in Chapter 8. It's been necessary to recognize its significance here because the amount of fiber that people eat probably reduces the amount of harm that fat can do. In fact, the reason that many epidemiological studies of the relationship between fat and cancer seem to contradict each other may be that they didn't take into account the amount of fiber that people were eating.

Another reason may be that "fat" is not simply fat.

Three Kinds of Fat

There are three types: saturated, monounsaturated, and polyunsaturated. The categories are determined by the chemical structure—the degree of "saturation" depends on structure (see page 167). Closely related to the saturated fats is a waxy material called *cholesterol*.

Cholesterol has gotten a lot of bad publicity, but it's important to health—the basic building material of steroid hormones. The body makes cholesterol all the time—using and recycling it endlessly. When too much cholesterol is in the blood, it clings to the interior walls of blood vessels, causing bottlenecks that result in cardiovascular disease, heart attacks, and strokes. Cholesterol is a necessary but undependable ally.

Cutting back on the amount of cholesterol we eat in our food may not make a very great difference in the cholesterol levels in our blood—but that little bit of difference may be crucial.

What is the relation between cholesterol and cancer?

One of the great truths unearthed by epidemiology is that countries which have high rates of colorectal cancer also have high rates of heart disease and also have high per capita consumption of fats!

Analysis of per capita fat intake in twenty industrialized countries shows a strong direct correlation between the amount of all the fat eaten by an individual and the mortality rate of colon cancer.

But this type of statistical analysis is based on the total amount of fat that a *country* eats, then dividing it arithmetically by the total population of the country, or the total number of cases of a particular type of cancer. It's something like dividing up the national debt into how much is owed by each man, woman, and child.

But real people tend to eat more, or less, than the national average—and it's real people who get cancer.

When individuals are studied, some remarkable facts emerge. The cholesterol levels of colon-cancer patients measured at the time of diagnosis were found to be *lower* than expected. Why? It could be that the cancers themselves were the cause— perhaps the malignancy requires cholesterol for growth, or causes some biochemical imbalance in the body that leads, indirectly, to lower cholesterol. On the other hand, maybe the cancer begins more readily when cholesterol levels are low to begin with.

In the massive Framingham Heart Study, men with low cholesterol levels developed more cancers of the colon—and some other sites—than men with normal or high levels. But this wasn't seen in women in the study.

The 7,961-man Honolulu Heart Study seemed to suggest a trade-off. Among the 598 men who died during the nine years of the study, high serum cholesterol was directly associated with death from heart disease, but inversely associated with deaths from cancer, especially cancers of the esophagus, colon, liver, lung, and leukemia. The higher the serum cholesterol, the lower their risk of these malignancies.

Colon Cancer or Heart Disease?

What's going on? Must we choose between eating rich foods and dying of coronary heart disease or stroke, on the one hand, or disciplining ourselves into a low-fat life and dying of colon cancer?

I asked Dr. Selwyn A. Broitman, an expert on gastrointestinal cancers at Boston University Medical School, and a member of the NAS committee.

"I suppose you need more studies to see whether low cholesterol is a cause or an effect of colon cancer," I ventured.

"You got it," said Dr. Broitman, a man who conveys the feeling that he thinks his work is the most fascinating in the world, and as he goes on in his down-to-earth Boston accent, you find yourself drawn into that fascination.

"But we already know lots of interesting things about cholesterol and cancer. One is that in countries where the diet is high in fat *and* high in cholesterol, lots of people will develop colon cancer and lots will develop heart disease.

"But they aren't the same people!"

Investigators have searched around the world for patients with *both* coronary heart disease *and* cancer of the colon, and have been able to find only twenty-three. Interestingly, all were on diets designed to *lower* their cholesterol.

We differ vastly in the way our bodies handle cholesterol, Dr. Broitman told me. In the United States, the mean level in adults is 210 milligrams of cholesterol per 10 milliliters of blood, and the range is from about 150 to 275, much too high, says the American Health Foundation, who argue that the ideal mean is about 160.

People with cholesterol levels over 300 have a high risk of heart disease. By restricting their intake of cholesterol and other fats in the diet, they can bring the serum levels down, but not very much, as a rule.

And there are people with serum levels of 200 to 220. "For most of these people, no matter how much cholesterol they eat, the serum levels don't budge much," says Dr. Broitman.

The extra cholesterol these people eat never gets into the blood at all, says Dr. Broitman. It's *excreted*. Cholesterol is eliminated with the other fat-soluble wastes, in the stools, since it can't be flushed away in the urine.

"Is cholesterol a problem for some people because it hangs around in the blood and clogs the vessels, and for others because it's constantly excreted?" I wondered. Then the significance dawned on me. "Oh, I see. If cholesterol is excreted in the stools, then the intestine is exposed to cholesterol all the time. Does that mean cholesterol may be causing colon cancer?"

"Could be," said Dr. Broitman. "There is a large group of people who eat lots of cholerestol who probably don't develop coronary heart disease, since they excrete much of it

73

through the colon. Maybe that is the group of people who are developing colon cancer!''

Dr. Broitman added that about twenty-five percent of the population isn't able to excrete cholesterol efficiently. Their moderate blood levels (220 to 250) shoot up when their cholesterol intake is increased. For them, eating a lot of cholesterol puts them in danger of heart disease, not colon cancer, since the substance backs up in their blood.

When you eat a food that contains cholesterol, a complex chain of events takes place. Digestive juices in the stomach break foods down into smaller chemical parts, and cholesterol is altered to form compounds called bile acids. In the colon, hordes of different kinds of intestinal bacteria busily break down the food components even further, and some types of bacteria can act on bile acids to form cancer promoters.

As we've seen in experimental animals, cancer promoters require repeated opportunities to act on cells; a single exposure doesn't cause a tumor to burst forth.

If a person is a cholesterol excreter, his colon is constantly exposed to promoters formed from bile acids. The situation resembles, in fact, a cleverly designed experiment to see how well a person's tissues stand up to regular, low doses of carcinogens.

For at least three or four decades, most people's tissues stand up very well to the never-ending challenges.

For this reason, as Dr. Walter Mertz says, you can go on a cholesterol spree now and again without ill effect, providing— and this is important—you give your colon a chance to recover from the resulting dose of promoters.

That is why, after a grand dinner with filet mignon, elegant sauces and puffy little cheese things at cocktail time, I treat myself to a few days of a very low-fat, high-fiber meals.

Polyunsaturated Fats and Cancer

If you think that cholesterol is the only greasy villain, pay attention. Since the 1940's, it's been known that in experimental animals, high-fat diets heighten responsiveness to standard carcinogens. This holds true for radiation-induced tumors as well as those elicited chemically.

In the past few years, researchers have been looking at the

effects of *specific* types of fats, and the distressing news is that polyunsaturated fats are no longer unquestioned heroes.

The NAS committee noted that polyunsaturated fat—usually in the form of corn oil—speeded up carcinogen-induced tumors in animals, even as it reduced cholesterol levels in the serum.

The cancer-enhancing effect is particularly noticeable when the total amount of fat in the diet is very low—five percent of calories. On higher-fat diets, it doesn't seem to matter whether the fat comes from saturated sources like coconut oil or lard, or from polyunsaturated oils.

Possibly, by clearing the blood of cholesterol, polyunsaturated fats increase the amount of cholesterol excreted through the colon. Maybe the excess cholesterol leads to an increase in bile acids. These may work either directly, as cancer promoters, on the lining of the colon, or they may be transformed by the intestinal bacteria into compounds that do the actual harm.

Or perhaps the polyunsaturates act, in a setting where not much fat of any kind is around, in some completely different way to encourage cancer.

Nobody is ready to draw firm conclusions yet, but the outlines are clear.

How Much Fat—and What Kinds Should We Eat?

The NAS committee agreed that the present level of fat in the American diet is too high. The official estimate is that forty percent of our calories come from fat, but most experts consider that estimate conservative, and all agree that some individuals eat much, much more fat.

The committee's interim dietary recommendation is that we cut back on our fat calories to thirty percent. Most members I've spoken with say that a thirty percent level is pretty liberal, and hope people will cut down still further.

The goal of reducing fat calories to thirty percent was chosen largely because it was felt that a greater proposed reduction would be too drastic and people wouldn't try to follow the recommendation at all.

But the American Health Foundation's vice-president, Dr. John H. Weisburger, thinks that we could bring the level down to twenty percent—"And in their own self-interest, people ought to try," he says.

The evidence that polyunsaturated fats encourage cancers in animals, and that cholesterol and high levels of saturated fats add to the risk of colon, breast, and other cancers in humans, is provocative but not quite solid enough, as yet, to tell the public to cut out one type of fat or another, the committee decided, after much deliberation.

Going on the available evidence, the NAS committee says that for the time being we should plan our food so that a third of our fat comes from polyunsaturated sources, a third from monounsaturated, and a third from saturated fats.

The committee's word on fat predictably did not sit well with the segments of the food industry involved in producing high-fat foods. There were cries of "Not proven!" which sounded, to some, like the howls emanating from the tobacco industry whenever a new study confirms the cigarette–lung-cancer link.

More fairly, the Meat Institute raised the point that only two years earlier, the Food and Nutrition Board of the National Academy of Sciences had stated in *its* report that "there is no basis for making recommendations to modify the proportions of these macronutrients [i.e., fat] in the American diet at this time."

Yet here was another body from the very same academy, announcing that a hefty reduction was in order. I was curious myself about this apparent 180-degree shift, so I asked the NAS project director, Dr. Sushma Palmer, about it.

"The Food and Nutrition Board reviewed only a small part of the whole scientific literature on the subject, whereas the Committee on Diet, Nutrition, and Cancer read, and took into account, *every published article*," Dr. Palmer told me. The sheer weight of evidence was several times greater for the 1982 report.

Furthermore, during the two-year interim, several important epidemiological studies were completed, helping to define the connections between fat and both colon and breast cancers more clearly. Better evidence, and more of it, justified their firmer stance, the committee concluded.

Well, why not cut out *all* fat, altogether?

That would be unhealthy in its own way and would eventually lead to serious malnourishment. Dietary fat includes *essential fatty acids* necessary to healthy life. The most important is linoleic acid, which maintains the membranes that shape the cells of the body. Other essential fatty acids are important in regulating the excretion of cholesterol, and serve as the raw materials for prostaglandins, thromboxanes, and prostacyclins—all tremendously important chemicals that regulate many physiological processes. Altogether, about one to two percent of our daily calories should be coming from essential fatty acids (which we get from meats, vegetables, and vegetable oils).

Don't worry about whether your diet is fat-deficient. Fats are inescapable. Cut way back, in every way you can, trim your meat, drink low-fat milk, take advantage of every dietary trick in the later chapters, and you still won't go short of fat.

There's a full gram of fat in a cup of *raisins*, for heaven's sake!

The intelligent course is to get the most possible enjoyment out of minimal amounts of fat in your everyday diet, and have some intensively low-fat strategies to follow when you want to compensate for a banquet or a barbecue.

8
Friendly Fiber

If fat is a slimy scoundrel, slipping around in our blood and innards in various sinister forms, then fiber is a plain, steady, down-home friend, doing an unglamorous job with total efficiency and dedication. Fiber asks for no credit, just for a chance to help.

Fiber is a catchall term for a dozen or more known chemical compounds that serve as the cellular skeletons of plants. Fruits, vegetables, and whole grains all contain fiber of several kinds.

Chemically, fibers are carbohydrates, similar to sugars and starches, but these are indigestible by humans, and are, strictly speaking, nonnutritive. So far as we're concerned, fiber is calorie-free—you can oxidize it in your fireplace, but you can't burn it in your body.

Till recently, nutritionists thought that while fiber, or "roughage," had a healthy laxative effect, it served no higher purpose and was, so to speak, just passing through. The same results can be obtained faster with a doze of herbal tea or milk of magnesia.

Fiber's indigestibility led early nutrition researchers to pass it by in favor of the more dramatic nutrients, like vitamins. A deficiency of a vitamin leads to an identifiable disease like pellagra or scurvy; a fiber deficiency leads to nothing worse than simple constipation—or so it was thought.

As life supposedly got better, people ate less and less fiber. Breads and porridges, the ancient whole-grain mainstays of all but the very rich, were replaced by meat and other fatty foods that had been special-occasion treats for most people.

To make flour white and "refined," millers sifted away

the hulls and husks from wheat. Fresh fruit, once a seasonal blessing and a rare luxury the rest of the year, became so commonplace that many people have ceased to regard an orange or fresh pineapple or even a mango as anything special at all. When we want a treat, it's more often ice cream or a Twinkie.

Westerners come from a long heritage of high-toned, low-fiber eating. European travelers in the nineteenth and early twentieth centuries pitied primitive people in Africa, Asia, and South America whom they saw subsisting on rice, millet, and strange vegetables. To good Victorians, everyday, wholesome food meant one thing—*flesh*. Mutton or goose or the roast beef of England, with desserts of creamy custard and charlotte russe. And everything was pounded and ground to a monotone of smoothness and refinement—no wonder the cuisine of foreign lands seemed coarse.

Fiber—often referred to as *crude* fiber—acquired old-fashioned, ugly, uncivilized connotations. It's what we've spent centuries trying to get away from. It's what *animals* eat!

But these days, the world's most sophisticated scientists are falling all over each other to get at the subtle mysteries of this primitive stuff.

How Fiber Helps

Fiber seems to rescue us daily while dietary fat and passing carcinogens are doing their best to do us in.

Fiber's laxative effect ensures that, if we eat enough of it, nothing bad can remain inside the digestive tract for very long. The effect on cancer risk can be profound.

Many Americans have a bowel movement only every other day or so. The Finns, with their very high fiber diet, have, on the average, a bowel movement daily, sometimes *two*. Their colon cancer incidence is much lower than ours.

The stools of high-fiber eaters are light and bulky; those of people who eat very little fiber are small and dense. Any poisons or carcinogens in a nonfiber-eater's diet are concentrated in the colon and may remain for days, but a diet containing plenty of fiber dilutes harmful substances so that the lining of the colon is exposed to lower concentrations. Fiber is firm and tough, and keeps its shape despite all the churning and chemical activity taking place in the gastrointestinal tract. Fiber's bristly consistency gives the intestinal lining a gentle scrub as it moves through, preventing cancer-promoting agents or other dangerous chemicals from lingering and building up. The housekeeping chores your colon needs can't be performed by a refined, civilized diet with its low fiber content.

Finally, fiber encourages the growth of intestinal bacteria. Dr. Bengt Gustafsson of the Karolinska Institute of Stockholm has been studying the ways of these microscopic organisms. As members of the plant kingdom, they are described sometimes as "intestinal flora."

"These bacteria grow best when they have something to cling to, and the more surfaces there are in their environment, the more opportunity the intestinal flora have to be fruitful and multiply," says Dr. Gustafsson. "Now, fiber comes from plants, and if you look at a plant under a microscope you see that it's made up of a series of microscopic boxes—all made of fiber.

"By the time they reach the colon, those boxes have been broken open, and the intestinal flora can swarm inside and outside, multiplying energetically."

Dr. Denis P. Burkitt, and his British colleague, Dr. Hugh Trowell, observed many years ago that colon cancer—and a host of other digestive ailments—were unheard of in primitive African people on high-fiber diets. At his own surgical clinic, Dr. Burkitt recalls, he performed only a handful of appendectomies, mostly on Europeans.

"So-called civilized people spend millions of pounds on laxatives and digestive remedies, but people in the Third World who are desperately poor go through life without knowing what constipation, hemorrhoids, gallbladder disease, or colon cancer are!" says Dr. Burkitt. "It's because they eat the fiber and bran that civilization tells us we should throw away."

Cancer investigators don't agree unanimously with Dr. Burkitt. They point out that while his observations about the lack of colon cancer in undeveloped countries are insightful, they only point up the need for more precise studies to determine the *nature* of the link between high fiber and a low incidence of colon cancer.

It could be that Third World people die of infectious diseases or accidents before colon cancers have a chance to develop. Maybe the high-fiber/low-colon-cancer association is just a variation on Richard Peto's playful fantasy that cancer is caused by telephones.

Epidemiological studies examining the proposition that high-fiber diets protect against colon cancer have sometimes supported Dr. Burkitt's contentions, and sometimes contradicted them.

The NAS committee examined all the evidence and discovered that studies lumping all the types of fiber together have masked the possibility that particular kinds may have a more protective effect than others. There are, after all, about a dozen different kinds of fiber. "Correlations have been based primarily on estimates of fiber intake obtained by grouping foods according to their fiber content," the committee reported.

In a study of fiber intake in various parts of Great Britain that at first found no correlation between fiber intake and mortality from colorectal cancer, the investigators took a more detailed look. They determined that there *was* a connection between low colon-cancer incidence and high consumption of a single type of fiber known as the *pentosan fraction*, found in whole grains and in vegetables other than potatoes.

With important evidence that the pentosan fraction, rather than all fiber collectively, may be responsible for protection against colon cancer, a blanket endorsement of fiber in general could send people in a lot of wrong directions.

At the same time, nobody is ready to say that the pentosan fraction deserves credit for *all* the good work that fiber does.

"We're just at the beginning of our understanding of fiber," sayd the Department of Agriculture's Dr. Walter Mertz. "There are many types of substances in what we call fiber, and they all have different effects. So the report touched on fiber rather lightly and our recommendations were cautious."

The committee could afford to be cautious because the balanced, varied, moderate diet they endorse is de facto replete with fiber. If you eat the fruits, vegetables, and whole grains necessary to get the vitamins, minerals, and trace nutrients you need, you can't help getting the fiber you need, too.

Why not *add* fiber, in a concentrated form? A few years

ago, commercial bakeries introduced new kinds of bread, made with white flour plus additional fiber. The fiber is tasteless and colorless and does nothing to change the flavor or texture of the "enriched" white bread.

"Those 'added fiber' foods show how far human beings can go when we overdo things," exclaimed Dr. Mertz. "First, we take out the fiber which is in there naturally. Bad enough. Then we think, perhaps there was something good in that fiber we took out, so we put part of it back in. Why do that? Why add that sawdust? Why not leave the natural fiber in there in the first place?"

"It doesn't make much sense," I agreed, but Dr. Mertz had more to say.

"And another thing," he continued. "I'd need very strong evidence to be convinced that it's *safe* to put in nonnutritive fiber that wasn't there in the first place. I don't see any such evidence, and I wouldn't touch the stuff!"

Another word of warning. Like any good thing, fiber can be overdone. Too much of it, nutritionists say, can interfere with the absorption of minerals in the intestine. How much is too much? It's not known. But if you're eating a balanced, varied, moderate diet, paying special attention to fiber but not consuming it to the exclusion of healthy nonfibrous foods, you'll probably be just fine.

9

Two Clear Warnings

The NAS Dietary Guidelines include two cautions about specific items which play a more important role in the lives of some people than others. If you don't drink alcohol, or do so only rarely, and if you dislike salty foods, or avoid them altogether in order to keep your sodium intake down, then these warnings won't make any difference in your personal habits of eating and drinking.

Alcohol

The evidence that heavy drinking, especially when combined with smoking, increases the risks of certain types of cancer is very strong, indeed. But how much risk is involved in the regular consumption of moderate amounts of liquor, beer, wine, and other alcoholic beverages isn't clear at all. The epidemiological studies that led the NAS committee to urge that alcoholic beverages should be used lightly, if at all, were conducted in groups of people who drank to *excess*. But the evidence was strong enough in the NAS committee's view to warrant an explicit, sobering recommendation.

In one of these studies—one of the very first to be conducted anywhere—it was shown, in 1910, that chronic absinthe drinkers in France had an appallingly high incidence of cancer of the esophagus. Since then, this cancer has been linked solidly to the heavy drinking of whiskey and of various potent local brews such as maize liquor in tribal Africa, apple brandy in Normandy, and the rice liquors of China and Japan.

Alcohol abuse is also strongly associated with primary cancers of the liver. These are known as hepatomas; so far as is known, alcohol has nothing to do with metastatic cancer that spreads to the liver from primary cancers arising in other tissues.

Alcohol also increases the carcinogenic effects of cigarette smoke on the upper digestive and respiratory tracts. Heavy drinkers who are also heavy smokers have a much higher incidence of cancers of the mouth, throat, pharynx, head, and neck than either nonsmoking drinkers or nondrinking smokers.

What's in This Drink?

Ethyl alcohol, or ethanol, is the chemical term for the particular type of alcohol present in alcoholic beverages. The proportion of alcohol varies with the strength of the particular beverage—water usually accounts for half the volume or more. Many beverages also contain sugar. In addition, all alcoholic beverages contain minute amounts of substances which give a drink its characteristic flavor, bouquet, and color; these are known as *congeners*. The deeper the color, the more intense the taste and aroma, the more congeners a drink contains.

Congeners give alcoholic beverages their distinctive personalities, and they're surrounded with a veil of mystery. The mystique is partly genuine, for these complicated organic compounds haven't all been defined, but some of the secrecy is a matter of commercial advantage. The religious orders who create pricey liqueurs like Chartreuse, Strega, and Benedictine guard their sacred blends of herbs and spices, and the more worldly makers of whiskeys, beers, and liquors of all kinds are equally dedicated to keeping the trade secrets of their flavorings, aromatics, and coloring agents.

But some scientists look with suspicion on congeners. It's not known whether congeners cause cancer, since most have never been identified. The question concerns nutrition expert Dr. George V. Mann, of Vanderbilt University, deeply enough for him to advise his patients who drink to avoid any alcoholic drink that isn't crystal clear, limiting them to vodka, gin, light rum, and white wine.

Animal studies show nearly everything alcoholic that people drink contains some highly suspect substances. These include our old friends the nitrosamines, plus polycyclic aromatic hydrocarbons, and even asbestos fibers, which can leach into wine, beer, and gin from filters used in the processing of some brands.

Putting congeners in the context of what's known about carcinogenesis, it's clear that if any of these substances are promoters, the danger would come from drinking appreciable amounts of the *same* kind of liquor, year after year. This is probably what happens with groups of people whose drinking is limited, by geography or economics, to the local traditional drink, like the groups mentioned at the beginning of this section.

Common sense would suggest that if we're going to drink much alcohol, it would be smart to *vary* our choices, just as we should do with our foods.

Apart from any carcinogenic effects of congeners, the ethanol in alcoholic beverages has indirect effects which may contribute to cancer. Excessive drinking, of course, damages the liver, causing scarring, or *cirrhosis*. When the damaged liver tries to heal itself, something may go terribly wrong with the healing process, leading to cancer of the liver.

Alcohol is also an efficient solvent, and it may act as a convenient means of transport for carcinogens that don't dissolve in water. As a result, initiators and promoters insoluble in water, which normally flow past the epithelial cells lining the esophagus and mouth like drops of oil in a watery salad dressing, get a free ride into those cells when they are dissolved in alcohol. That may be one reason for the high incidence of mouth and esophageal cancers in heavy drinkers.

Heavy drinkers tend to be in big nutritional trouble, which may add to their overall chances of developing cancer. An alcohol abuser may consume twenty-five to fifty percent of his calories as alcohol, calories which bring no nutritional value. To keep slim, they skip meals and subsist on "liquid lunches," which is not difficult since alcohol is an appetite suppressant. And someone who is drinking a lot may simply forget to eat.

What nutrients a heavy drinker does take in are depleted by the impact of alcohol on the body. To handle ethanol, the liver has to use up thiamine and niacin, two of the B vitamins, and alcohol blocks the absorption of two others, folacin and vitamin B_{12}. The B vitamins are profoundly important to the immune system, as we'll see in Chapter 10. Finally, with its very efficient diuretic effects, alcohol washes away water-soluble nutrients.

But alcohol in light or moderate quantities has not, thus far, been shown to have any carcinogenic effects, and therefore the NAS committee urges moderation, not abstinence.

Heavily Salt-Cured Foods

People who eat large quantities of heavily smoked, salt-cured, or salt-pickled foods face the very real threat of stomach cancer.

"Salting things down" is an ancient practice, which works because bacteria and other microorganisms which cause foods to spoil cannot live in an environment that is too salty. Before the days of refrigeration, salt was the best way to preserve meat or fish until it was needed. Sometimes, particularly with ham and bacon, a brine made with sodium nitrite was used. Sometimes the foods were smoked, as well.

These preservatives eliminate the immediate danger of potentially lethal diseases like botulism and other kinds of food poisoning. But as refrigeration improved, these old-fashioned food-preserving methods declined. When the change was introduced, around 1900, the incidence of stomach cancer, once a major killer in the U.S., started to decline.

The traditional salt-curing methods have been largely abandoned, even for foods that many people consider "salt-cured." The one exception is "country-cured" meats like Smithfield ham. These are so mouth-puckeringly salty that most of us eat them only sparingly, if at all.

The "old-fashioned" smokehouse flavor of most sausage, ham, and bacon available at your supermarket comes from soaking these meats in smoke-flavored solutions, or even injecting them with it. Either way, the meat does not acquire the dark-brown glaze of smoky particles that develops during long-term hanging in a smokehouse. Genuine smoking laces the food with polycyclic aromatic hydrocarbons, many of which are known mutagens, and at least two of which are potent carcinogens in laboratory animals.

The preservatives used in processed meats can form nitrosamines. Nitrites, principally saltpeter, and nitrates used in processed meats (bologna, salami, cold cuts, ham, bacon, and sausage) can, under these circumstances, combine with amino acids to form nitrosamines. This can happen in the food itself, but it happens on a much grander scale within your stomach.

On the other hand, nitrites and nitrates prevent the propagation of bacteria, they impart the rosy color we've come to expect, and add a subtle edge of flavor.

During the 1970's, the cancer-causing potential of nitrosamines came to public attention. In 1980, the FDA decided that there wasn't enough evidence to justify a ban on sodium nitrite, since not one cause of human cancer has been traced to nitrosamines, nitrates, or nitrites in foods. However, the U.S. Department of Agriculture ordered the meat industry to eliminate these preservatives entirely from some products and to reduce the amounts used in others. Better safe than sorry. Now ascorbic acid (vitamin C) is used widely instead.

So, unless you make hot dogs, ham, and cold cuts your main meats, you needn't worry much.

Overseas, however, huge quantities of traditional salt-cured, salt-pickled, and smoked foods continue to be eaten in some countries. Most that I've sampled are too pronounced in flavor for my taste, and probably for most other Americans.

But in some places, the people eat these foods at a great rate. In some parts of China, pickled vegetables are a dietary staple; there stomach cancer is a major killer. In Japan, the traditional cuisine requires salt pickled vegetables and fish—and has been linked to the high Japanese incidence of stomach cancer.

In the Scandinavian countries, the affinity for heavily salted and pickled foods amounts to a passion. A meal without *some* kind of seriously salty food—usually fish in some form—is apparently unthinkable to Swedes, Norweigians, Icelanders, and Danes.

I learned this one morning at the lavish help-yourself *fruktost* table at a Stockholm hotel. The sight of the beautifully arranged sliced cheeses and cold meats, the vast assortment of crisp flatbreads and hearty whole-grain breads began to wake me up, and when I spied the crocks of fruit jams and preserves, my mouth began to water. Some extraordinarily good berries grow in the northern countries which aren't found elsewhere; they're turned into preserves of luxurious flavor and brilliant color.

A friendly Swede pointed to some interesting looking rose-colored stuff in one of the crocks. "Try some, it's really good," he said. "No Swedish breakfast is complete without it."

So I slathered some on a slice of rich whole-grain bread. But when I bit into it—what an experience! It was intensely salty and strongly *fishy*. Not bad for a cocktail canape, but not the sort of thing Americans are used to for breakfast.

"Um, it certainly is *Swedish*," I said as politely as I could.

"Ja-ja, it's Swedish," said my companion, who helped himself to more. Later, I found that the rosy delicacy is called *löjrom*—fish roe cured in salt. A kind of caviar, you might say. But our sissified American palates aren't attuned to caviar for breakfast, or highly salted foods as a dietary mainstay—and a good thing, too.

Along with salted fish, Scandinavians, particularly Icelanders, consume a lot of home-smoked foods, particularly smoked trout and smoked mutton. In Iceland, where the consumption of these foods is highest, the stomach cancer incidence soars.

On the other hand, Icelandic sailors have a much lower rate of stomach cancer than their stay-at-home friends and relatives, possibly because they may eat more fresh fruits and vegetables. Their ships take on these foods when they put in at foreign ports.

Japanese studies show that fresh foods, like milk, and western vegetables, like lettuce and celery which are eaten raw, help to protect against stomach cancer. Many of them contain vitamin C, which could be acting as an antioxidant to protect against the nitrosamines formed from other foods in the stomach.

In the U.S., we eat rather modest amounts of truly smoked and heavily salt-cured foods. There are only small amounts of nitrites and nitrates in our cured and processed meats, which we often eat with coleslaw, tomatoes, and carrot sticks. As a nation, we are already doing a lot of things right to prevent stomach cancer, and our declining incidence of the disease seems to bear it out.

Nevertheless, the NAS committee felt bound to warn people against eating these foods in excess.

"Looking at the *world* picture, these foods present a big problem," says Dr. Broitman. "The data we based our recommendations on come from overseas, but they're relevant to the ethnic groups who've moved to this country and kept their traditional methods of cooking and preserving foods—the Japanese and Filipinos in Hawaii, for example.''

The NAS committee's recommendation is that ''the consumption of food preserved by salt-curing (including salt-pickling) be minimized.'' But chances are that our own likes and dislikes are already minimizing our intake quite effectively. I don't think you would care much for *löjrom* for breakfast, either.

10
Mighty Micronutrients

Some of our most important allies in our struggle to stay healthy are the ones we require in the smallest amounts. These are little giants—vitamins, minerals, and trace elements—which are inordinately powerful and utterly necessary to life. Every day, we need about half a teaspoonful of these *micronutrients*.

Vitamins

The thirteen recognized vitamins are all organic (carbon-based) chemical compounds with recognized chemical structures as familiar to those who work with them as H_2O is to a basic-chemistry student.[1]. Vitamins define themselves, in a way, by their absence. A diet devoid of a particular vitamin results eventually in a specific cluster of symptoms, a *deficiency disease*.

Too little vitamin A and a person develops night blindness and skin problems, too little vitamin C and he gets the deficiency called scurvy.

---

[1]There are 13 recognized vitamins. Their alphabetical designations are confusing, since some, first thought to be single chemical compounds, have been found to be several separate substances with important, independent functions. Other vitamins, identified by a single letter, are really groups of closely related chemicals, or different compounds that have the same biological activity in the body. The roster as it stands today:

Vitamin A (retinoic acid)
Vitamin B_1 (thiamine)
Vitamin B_6 (pyridoxine,
   pyridoxal, and pyridoxamine)
Vitamin B_{12} (the cobalamins)
Vitamin C (ascorbic acid)
Vitamin D (ergocalciferol
   or cholecalciferol)
Vitamin E (alpha-tocopherol)

Vitamin K (phyoolquinone or
   menaquinone)
Riboflavin (formerly B_2)
Niacin (formerly vitamin B_3)
Folacin (also called folic
   acid; once thought to be a
   B vitamin)
Pantothenic acid
Biotin

But it's apparent that vitamins do much more in the body than stave off deficiency diseases.

For at least one vitamin—vitamin A—there is enough evidence to support the idea that it acts against the development of cancer for the NAS committee to recommend that we emphasize the dark-green and deep-yellow vegetables containing sources of vitamin A.

There is evidence that vitamin C, too, has some cancer-protective effect. The committee urges us to include in our daily diet foods that contain vitamin C, such as citrus fruits. We'll examine the evidence concerning vitamins and cancer in a moment.

Micronutrients also include minerals. We need seven minerals in fairly large quantities: calcium, phosphorus, magnesium, potassium, sulfur, sodium, and chloride. These are known as the *macro*minerals. We need as many as sixteen more *micro*minerals, in much smaller quantities.

Unlike vitamins, which are big, fancy molecules with lots of carbon, hydrogen, and oxygen atoms, minerals are simpler inorganic substances which can enter the body as ingredients in smaller chemical compounds. Inside the body, the mineral breaks free of its carrier compound and gets busy.

Vitamins and Cancer

The NAS committee's advice to eat fruits (especially citrus fruits), dark-green and dark-yellow vegetables, cruciferae (cabbage and its cousins), plus whole-grain cereal products, is designed to ensure that people will take in the *full* range of micronutrients they need, for general good health and for lowering their risks of cancer.

The evidence is strong and well supported that some of the micronutrients, and perhaps other, less publicized constitutents of food, have a more direct action against cancer than just maintaining normal well-being.

Vitamin A and Cancer

The most talked about, and perhaps the most potent, is vitamin A—also known as retinoic acid. (The name is related to *retina*, the filmy curtain at the back of the eyeball where vitamin A plays a crucial role in vision.) When a person is deficient in vitamin A, one of the first symptoms is a growing inability to adapt to dim light (night blindness). Prolonged deficiency, especially in young children, damages the eye tissues and can result in blindness.

In its retinol form, vitamin A is what chemists call an alcohol. It exists in fish, liver, dairy products, meats, and egg yolks. It can also be made, in the body, from various *provitamin* compounds, as it's needed. The best known of these is *beta-carotene*, which, predictably, comes from carrots. Cantaloupe, broccoli, spinach, and all the dark-green and dark-yellow vegetables contain the golden provitamin.

For every six molecules of beta-carotene you take in, your body makes one molecule of vitamin A.

On the face of it, it would seem that a daily vitamin A pill would be the most efficient way of getting the retinol you need, but human nutrition is seldom that simple. Like some of the minerals discussed earlier, too much retinol can be a decidedly bad thing for you—causing skin abnormalities, blurred vision, jaundice, hair loss, and bone deformities if you take too much for too long. Vitamin A is powerful stuff, not something you can dose yourself with casually, expecting only good to result.

It is safe to eat lots of foods containing beta-carotene, however. The worst that can happen is that your skin can turn an odd orangey color if you eat too much, but while this condition may draw some puzzled glances, it's harmless, so far as anyone knows, and goes away after one stops eating excessive amounts of beta-carotene.

Several years ago, Dr. Michael B. Sporn of the National Cancer Institute began discussing experiments he and his team had done which showed that 13-cis-retinoic acid (the vitamin A takes after being oxidized in the body) had some interesting effects on cancer cells in vitro. It seemed to be able to make them revert to normal.

Knowing that scientists can perform wonders in petri dishes with cells that have gotten special treatment, and knowing that these wonders aren't always translatable into human beings or even mice, I was skeptical that Dr. Sporn's work would mean much for patients with cancer, or even for people at risk.

But then, three years ago, Dr. Vincent T. DeVita, director

of the National Cancer Institute, told me quietly, "Keep your eye on beta-carotene. We're very excited about it!"

Sure enough, laboratory animals, epidemiological studies, and now ongoing studies in humans show that retinoic acid, and artificial analogues designed to have less toxicity, all seem to agree—vitamin A and its derivatives can sabotage the process of carcinogenesis.

That's a pretty good reason for excitement.

Now we know that during the development of the embryo, vitamin A is responsible for turning the immature, fast-dividing epithelial cells into the mature, specialized, nondividing cells that make up normal tissues. From conception to birth, it's important for the number of cells in the embryo to increase quickly, building up a complete baby that can survive in the outside world. The full-term baby needs a wide variety of cells that perform their assigned functions and do not divide very often; the embryo, whose needs are served by the mother's body, needs only to *grow*.

As time goes on, simple growth in the embryo becomes less important, and the need for operational organs, made up of mature cells, becomes paramount as birth approaches. *Differentiation*—the process we described in Chapter 3— begins to take place, signaled by chemical messengers.

One of them is vitamin A, which signals epithelial cells to differentiate, and, as we've said, the overwhelming majority of cancers originate in epithelial tissues.

The evidence shows consistently that deficiency in vitamin A increases laboratory animals' susceptibility to chemical carcinogenesis in the kinds of experiments described in Chapter 3. Stepping up the intake of vitamin A prevents or slows the development of these experimental tumors. When a *millimicrogram* of the vitamin is applied an hour before a powerful promoter is painted on, after the application of an equally potent initiator, hardly any tumors appear. (A millimicrogram is a *billionth* of a gram.)

Vitamin A doesn't always work so miraculously; if the initiator is given in multiple doses, it doesn't prevent the experimental tumors. And in some experimental situations, the number of tumors may be increased.

"You can't get up on a soapbox and say that retinoic acid *always* prevents cancer," says Dr. Roswell K. Boutwell.

"But in many cases, it does make cells on their way to becoming cancerous straighten up and fly right!"

And the absence of vitamin A makes it harder for cells to resist the effects of carcinogens.

"The epithelial cells in the respiratory tract don't differentiate properly in vitamin-A-deficient animals," says Dr. Boutwell. "And when a person is vitamin-A-deficient, a microscopic examination of his respiratory tract shows that the epithelial cells aren't mature, they're adolescent, with some similarities to cancer cells."

Epidemiological studies have focused, of course, on the *foods* people eat, and not on what, precisely, those foods contain. So when investigators perceive that the incidence of a particular cancer is lower among people who eat greater-than-average amounts of foods that contain vitamin A and beta-carotene (like carrots and eggs), they don't *know* for certain that the good work is being done by these components. It's a tempting assumption, since those forms of vitamin A are present in those foods, but there are other health-giving compounds in there as well, and maybe one of them deserves the credit.

Good News for Smokers

But diets supplying high levels of beta-carotene and vitamin A are linked, epidemiologically, with low risks of cancer of the esophagus, stomach, colon, rectum, prostate, and most dramatically, the lung!

And the really exciting part is that the protective effect of vitamin A seems strongest among *smokers*.

The great pioneer in this line of research, Dr. Erik Bjelke of the University of Bergen, Norway, measured the level of vitamin A in the diets of over 16,000 Norwegians and Americans. The Vitamin A index, as he calls it, tallies neatly with lung cancer risk.

"At all levels of smoking, the higher the vitamin A index, the *lower* the lung cancer risk," he told the Thirteenth International Cancer Congress in Seattle, Washington.

In my opinion, an intelligent smoker would spend as much money on carrots as on cigarettes! But even nonsmokers would do well to pay attention to the lessons of Dr. Bjelke's subjects and to those thousands of laboratory rats and mice.

If vitamin A and its relatives can protect epithelial tissues from the effects of horrendous carcinogens like those used in the lab and those in cigarette smoke, then it stands to reason that those protective compounds ought to be able to defend people from weaker, less understood carcinogens.

Dr. Bjelke and dozens of other investigators around the world are now looking for other, less obvious links between a high vitamin A index and a low incidence of other types of cancer. There are clues from other, smaller studies that need to be followed up. With epidemiology, just as with laboratory studies, a relatively modest effect can't be shown clearly unless a large number of people is studied.

The NAS committee, however, did not think it was necessary to wait around for additional evidence.

"The laboratory evidence shows that vitamin A itself, and many of the retinoids are able to suppress chemically induced tumors," their report concludes. "The epidemiological evidence is sufficient to suggest that foods rich in carotenes or vitamin A are associated with a reduced risk of cancer."

In effect, that means, "Eat your carrots. Bugs Bunny was right."

Vitamin C and Cancer

Vitamin C is another micronutrient that may help protect us against cancer, though the evidence concerning its helpful effects isn't nearly as extensive as the literature on vitamin A.

Nonetheless, the committee was convinced enough to urge us to consume plenty of foods containing this vitamin, otherwise known as ascorbic acid. The citrus fruits, heartily endorsed by the panel, as famous for their high vitamin C content.

Vitamin C is a potent antioxidant, quickly and harmlessly reacting with compounds that otherwise become electrophilic and perhaps carcinogenic. Vitamin C keeps them out of trouble, by defusing them chemically.

In the stomach, vitamin C firmly blocks the formation of the combination of nitrite compounds from some foods with amino acids from others.

A few years ago there was quite a flap about nitrosamines in food—principally in cured meats like frankfurters, ham, and bacon, and in some brands of beer. The public concern impelled meat packers and brewers to eliminate most of these preformed nitrosamines from their products. The brewers found that a single modification in the brewing process could eliminate nitrosamines, so nowadays, most major brands made in the U.S. are nitrosamine-free.

But then it was pointed out that people are much more efficient producers of nitrosamines than the meat or brewing industries ever were. A whole smorgasbord of nitrosamines can be assembled in your stomach minutes after you've eaten a good, healthy, balanced meal.

But nitrosamines can't form if enough ascorbic acid (or another antioxidant) is on the scene. Nitrite would really *rather* unite with vitamin C than with amino acids.

The solution is deliciously evident.

My own strategy is to eat something that contains vitamin C whenever I eat *anything*. Coleslaw with hot dogs, sliced tomatoes and onions on hamburger, lemon juice on plain broiled fish. I regard these vitamin-C-rich foods as necessities of life, an integral part of each meal.

Vitamin C's ability to prevent the formation of nitrosamines explains why research shows that people with cancer of the esophagus or stomach have a history of shying away from food containing this vitamin. In the absence of antioxidants, nitrosamines form unchecked, and the tender epithelial lining of the upper gastrointestinal areas is right there where the action is.

Laboratory studies also show that ascorbic acid can inhibit cancer in ways that have nothing to do with nitrosamine formation. The evidence is skimpy, admittedly, but it shouldn't be ignored.

Ascorbic acid added to normal cells kept alive in the test tube prevents carcinogens from turning these cells into cancer cells, even when the vitamin is added as long as twenty-three days later! Human leukemia cells kept alive by similar artificial means stop dividing when low concentrations of ascorbic acid are applied.

Of course, cells growing in vitro aren't the same as cells in a living person, and what happens in the lab may not duplicate what goes on inside us. So the possibility that some interesting anticancer events may be taking place beyond your digestive tract when you eat enough food containing vitamin C is not as yet nailed down. The scientists are working on it.

In the meantime, the clear lowering of the risk for stomach and esophageal cancers by ascorbic acid is enough, the NAS committee concluded, to warrant telling people who are healthy to pay special attention to fresh vegetables and fruits—especially the citrus family.

Some scientists suspect that the mysterious reduction in stomach cancer in the U.S. since the turn of the century may be due to refrigerated storage of foods that contain heat-sensitive vitamin C.

Other Vitamins and Cancer

What about the other vitamins?

It's shocking, but there wasn't enough evidence for the committee to draw any further conclusions about vitamins or make any additional recommendations about them. This is one reason why the committee warns against taking vitamin supplements—they can't say that too-high doses of vitamins won't upset the body's biochemical intricacy or even increase cancer risk!

Vitamin E has sometimes been shown to inhibit carcinogenesis in experimental animals—and sometimes it hasn't.

"Studies of the effect of vitamin E on carcinogenesis do not show severe or consistent inhibitory levels," the academy committee says in summary. "It is possible that vitamin E can inhibit, under certain conditions," the report speculates, but no one has yet devised a good means of testing the proposition.

As for epidemiology, the discipline offers no evidence that vitamin E has any effect at all on human cancer incidence. And, the committee observes, it may be hard to get any evidence. Vitamin E is present in so many foods (eggs, vegetable oils, whole grains, green leafy vegetables) that everybody gets pretty much the same amounts, whatever the dietary life-style. Epidemiologists would have to find two groups of people with substantially different intakes of the vitamin, and even epidemiologists, who are keen detectives, don't know where to look.

Vitamin E, like vitamin C, is an antioxidant and hence an inhibitor of nitrosamine formation. Vitamin E might protect

97

the stomach and esophagus when nitrites and amino acids are trying to get together. But, says the NAS committee, "There are no reports on the effect of this vitamin on nitrosamine-induced neoplasia," and, "the data are not sufficient to permit any firm conclusion to be drawn about the effect of vitamin E in humans."

What about the B vitamins?

A very few animal experiments have been performed to see whether various B vitamins affect the development of cancer. These are difficult questions to ask experimentally, let alone answer, for the B vitamins work with one another, and with other compounds, in relationships of such bureaucratic complexity that it's hard to fix responsibility. No one has begun to pinpoint the role of each of the B vitamins in coping with carcinogenesis.

Theoretically, the B vitamins might maintain the search-and-destroy patrol the immune system is thought to maintain. Despite the clever networks of anticarcinogenesis mechanisms, normal cells are subverted from time to time. It's speculated that certain white blood cells cruise the fluids of the body, looking for cancer cells that haven't had a chance to divide. The body's killer cells annihilate these young cancer cells, Pac-Man style, before they have a chance to cause trouble.

This concept of *immune surveillance* is attractive; there is some evidence that something of the kind goes on, but it hasn't been proved or worked out in detail. Any such process would require B vitamins to keep those patrolling cells strong and effective.

"It seems likely that major disruption of energy or carbohydrate metabolism by deficiencies of riboflavin or thiamine, vitamin B_2, and vitamin B_1, or disruption of normal cell replication by deficiencies . . . in vitamin B_{12} would affect immune surveillance," says the report.

This speculation would have to be proved in laboratory animals and buttressed by epidemiological findings that people with deficiencies in vitamins B_1, B_2, and B_{12} had a higher incidence of some cancer.

But the few laboratory studies on B vitamins and cancer are, in the view of the NAS committee, "inadequate," and, as with vitamin E, epidemiological studies are simply nonexistent.

And as for the other vitamins, the worldwide scientific literature has nothing whatever to say about their relationship, if any, to human cancer.

Minerals: Macro and Micro

The seven macrominerals are calcium, phosphorus, magnesium, potassium, sulfur, sodium, and chloride. You're probably not surprised to see calcium and phosphorus in the list: "they build strong bones and teeth," as some cereal commercials used to say. But, with all the bad press that salt has been getting, you may be surprised to see sodium. In fact, we couldn't live without sodium—220 milligrams, a twentieth of a teaspoon daily—to regulate the balance of water and chemicals in the fluid surrounding the cells. Within the cells, potassium performs this crucial regulatory function. For the system to work, potassium and sodium must be present in proper proportions.

The average American, however, consumes between five and eighteen grams daily, or between two and four teaspoonfuls, and most doctors consider the excess sodium a major cause of high blood pressure, or hypertension. (For a more detailed look at sodium's role in your daily diet, see page 173.)

Next come the microminerals, also called trace minerals or trace elements. The list is long but the requirements are tiny, measured in *micro*milligrams.

Nutritionists agree that we need iron, zinc, selenium, manganese, molybdenum, copper, iodine, chromium and flourine in these small amounts. We may also require nickel, cobalt, vanadium, silicon, tin, cadmium, and even arsenic.

Dr. Walter Mertz, of the U.S. Department of Agriculture, was a pioneer in determining the role of trace minerals in human nutrition. Over his desk hangs a chart of the periodic table of elements, hauntingly familiar to anybody who's ever taken a course in chemistry.

Dr. Mertz's chart is as big as a bedsheet and dominates the room.

"I look at it all day," he confessed to me. "There is something very interesting, *here,*" he said, indicating a series of elements in the middle of the table, and sneaking a long look at them as if he expected them to spell out the answer to some biochemical puzzle while he wasn't watching.

"Back in the 1940's and 1950's, when we made nutrient solutions to feed patients intravenously who couldn't eat regular food, the concoctions we prepared were not terribly pure. There were trace minerals in there by accident which we didn't know enough to put in by design.

"We didn't know it, but those contaminants were helping to keep the patients alive. It was only after we got too smart for ourselves and began to purify these solutions completely that we found our patients developing a whole flurry of deficiencies while living on nutrient solutions that were supposedly complete!"

Nowadays, intravenous feeding solutions are as carefully blended as the secret sauces of a famous chef. Instead of herbs and spices, they have a whole arsenal of micronutrients to augment the amino acids, essential fatty acids, and macronutrients. And just as with the artificial diets so carefully composed for laboratory animals, nutritionists fret over whether they have left something out.

Let's look at the microminerals and some of the roles they play:

Zinc is a vital constituent of at least a hundred enzymes in the human body, and plays a role in fending off disease, perhaps including cancer.

Selenium, which causes nervous-system toxicity, blindness, and death in amounts that are greater than infinitesimal, has a poorly understood but genuine anticancer effect. In parts of the United States with lower-than-average levels of selenium in soil and drinking water, the cancer rates are higher, and there are more deaths from heart attacks, too.

Fluorine helps maintain bones and teeth. *Manganese* is important to the central nervous system. *Cobalt* is a key part of vitamin B_{12} that cells require in order to replicate. *Molybdenum* may be unpronounceable, but it makes certain enzyme reactions possible.

Arsenic, in large doses a deadly poison, is—in tiny amounts—necessary to life. Animal studies show that without minute amounts of arsenic, the heart muscle deteriorates.

"And *chromium* is a cofactor for the normal function of insulin," said Dr. Mertz, who, I later learned, was the scientist who discovered that this shiny metal was good for something besides decorating the tail fins of 1950's Oldsmobiles.

Minerals and Cancer

Minerals may be relevant to cancer in two possible ways, which seem paradoxical and contradictory. The *absence* of a mineral, even one that's needed only in trace amounts, may wreak profound havoc in a person's life. Iron or copper deficiency can cause anemia. Iodine deficiency leads to goiter, and so on. It stands to reason that the faintest dose of some mineral on Dr. Mertz's periodic table might mean the difference between susceptibility and resistance to one step or another in carcinogenesis.

But the evidence falls short of what the NAS committee required. One big problem is that to spot the risks or benefits of a substance, epidemiologists need two groups of people who consume different amounts of that substance. With minerals, as with vitamin E, the intake varies little. And with *trace* minerals, differences are even harder to find. (Do some people ingest a full trace every day, while others squeak by with a trace of a trace?)

The committee examined the evidence for the nine minerals suspected of playing some role, good or bad, in human cancer—selenium, iron, copper, zinc, molybdenum, iodine, arsenic, cadmium, and lead—and for most, the phrase recurs, "the evidence does not permit any firm conclusions to be drawn." But there is some evidence—a trace or two—concerning several.

Iron. The strongest evidence about any of the minerals concerns iron. It's perhaps the least relevant, although, indirectly, it supports the contention that nitrosamines contribute to stomach cancer. There used to be an iron-deficiency disease called Plummer-Vinson syndrome—sometimes known as Paterson-Kelly—in certain parts of Sweden. People with the syndrome frequently developed cancers of the upper digestive tract. Now that improved nutrition has eliminated the deficiency, there are no new cases of this cancer-predisposing syndrome.

Dr. Selwyn Broitman and his Boston University team found

that in an iron-poor area of Colombia, in South America, iron deficiency permitted bacteria to colonize the stomachs of affected people. These bacteria reduced nitrates in the food to nitrites, leading to the formation of nitrosamines. These iron-deficient people have a high risk of stomach cancer.

Interestingly, patients with pernicious anemia—an iron-deficiency condition that leads to similar bacterially-produced nitrosamines in the stomach—also have increased risk of stomach cancer.

But neither Plummer-Vinson syndrome nor stomach cancer is a significant health problem in the U.S., and iron deficiency so far as is known plays no role in any of our major cancers.

Can iron be carcinogenic? Though clinical and epidemiological reports suggest that when people occupationally exposed to iron *inhale* large amounts of the metal in powder form, their cancer risk rises, the committee says there's no evidence to indicate that high levels of iron in your *diet* could add to your cancer risk.

Selenium. The importance of selenium first came to notice in the 1930's, when it was recognized as the cause of the disease of cattle known as the blind staggers. When cattle ate range grass containing toxic levels of selenium, their nervous systems were damaged severely and they often died.

Figuring that anything so dangerous to a cow could well pose threats to people, scientists began mapping the levels of selenium in soils, forages, and in human tissues, seeking to correlate these amounts with patterns of disease incidence.

When human per capita intake of selenium was calculated, and compared with cancer mortality rates in twenty countries, it became clear that the lower the selenium consumption, the greater the mortality from colon, rectum, pancreas, breast, ovary, and prostate cancers, all linked to fat consumption, and from bladder and skin cancers. The same also held true, in men only, for leukemia and cancer of the lung.

In 1973, it was discovered that selenium is part of an enzyme called glutathione peroxidase. This enzyme is an antioxidant, and because it acts on compounds derived from fats, the NAS committee says selenium "could well be involved in protecting against cancer induced by high intakes of fat.''

In the laboratory, selenium-deficient animals are extra-susceptible to chemically induced cancers; this susceptibility increased on diets supplemented with large amounts of poly-unsaturated fats.

Do you need selenium? Absolutely. Adults require 200 *micrograms* per day (a microgram is a *millionth part of a gram*). In the U.S., an ordinary, adequate diet provides that necessary amount, from foods such as seafood, whole-grain cereals, egg yolks, meat, poultry, milk, and garlic. *Selenium supplements are unnecessary, and they may be dangerous.*

Zinc. The NAS committee suggests that zinc may play a hero at some points in the cancer process and a villain at others. Zinc is essential to life, a constituent of more than a hundred enzymes, including some that are predominant in cell division, tissue repair, and growth. Zinc-deficient people have impaired reactions to the standard tests for immune-system efficiency, but just which link in a zinc-deprived immune system is the one that's weakened is not known.

Some studies suggest that high levels of zinc in the diet are associated with an *increase* in incidence of breast, stomach, and other cancers. Other research shows that patients with esophageal and respiratory cancers have lower-than-normal levels of zinc in their blood.

Too much zinc in the blood may force down the levels of selenium, which is, as we've seen, an anticancer factor. Zinc deficiency slows down tumor growth, for tumor cells, like normal cells, must have the mineral to stay alive. Cancer patients may have low zinc levels as a result of the disease, with the rapidly multiplying cancer cells plundering the body of its zinc reserves.

Perhaps zinc may help ward off cancer in the *early* stages, when few cancer cells are around, by keeping the immune system in tip-top order. Later on, when the disease has established itself and the cells are proliferating like mad, zinc, a key ingredient for cell division and growth, encourages them.

Studies at the University of Colorado found that if cereal makers put a little zinc in their products, zinc deficiency in cereal eaters would disappear.

But before we start writing letters to Cap'N Crunch, we'd best consider the NAS committee's astute and, at this point, unanswerable question: "Does zinc deficiency, believed to be widespread, especially among children, present a risk or provide protection against carcinogenesis?" In any event, the committee warns, don't take zinc supplements. With what little anyone knows, it would be difficult—and irresponsible—to say that the deficiency is either bad for us or good.

Should You Take Vitamin and Mineral Pills?

Biological systems, such as ourselves and rats or mice, are fastidious. We require a whole array of raw materials, but we must have them in the proper amounts. Too little, and we develop deficiencies; too much, and delicate mechanisms go crazy, like an overwound cuckoo clock.

For example, vitamin C, a vitamin which many people take in the form of supplemental tablets, can be both a hero and a villain in your body's biochemical drama. Vitamin C is essential to life, but too much of it can upset the body's mineral balance. "The vitamin greatly increases the absorption of iron, but it *interferes* with the absorption of copper, essential in forming red blood cells and making enzymes needed for respiration.

"And excessive amounts of vitamin C turn cancer-protective selenium compounds into metallic selenium, which isn't absorbed at all," says Dr. Mertz.

"This is one of the reasons why we counseled against taking vitamin and mineral supplements, and advised people to get their nourishment from the food they eat," Dr. Mertz says.

"We require lots of different nutrients, some in very small amounts, some perhaps in amounts that can't be detected. For thousands of years, we have been getting what we need from *foods*, not from tablets, because foods are full of many different kinds of nutrients and other substances.

"We can never be sure that we've discovered *all* the essential nutrients," Dr. Mertz told me. "You can put together a very complete artificial diet comprised of everything that we think humans require, but the diet cannot suffice if we've left out something we don't know about.

"Foods may well contain extremely important trace compounds which we don't even suspect are there!"

"A balanced, varied, moderate diet," I said to myself.

Dr. Mertz once again shifted his gaze to the big periodic table hanging over his desk.

11

Macronutrients: Where Calories Come From

11
Macronutrients: Where Calories Come From

The processes of life require energy, which comes from oxidizing, or burning, the food that the organism ingests. No living thing can get along without fuel, which is measured in units of heat, or *calories*. Our calories come from proteins, carbohydrates, and fats. These nutrients are the mainstays of the human diet, and because we need a fair amount of them, they are called *macronutrients*.

We've gotten the idea that calories are bad, but although excess calories lead to overweight and less-than-perfect health, we mustn't forget that calories are necessary to life.

Calories are also important because other nutrients we must have are inextricably bound up in calorie-providing foods. Except for those notorious "empty-calorie" foods like granulated sugar, everything we eat contains, in addition to its calories, some other health-giving substances. These are the vitamins, minerals, and other, less familiar chemicals which support good health. Among them (as later chapters discuss in detail) are some that help protect us against cancer.

Proteins, carbohydrates, and fats are broken down chemically into combustible pieces in the digestive tract and are absorbed by the body through the intestinal walls, then oxidized as fuel or stored in anticipation of later need. The form in which this surplus is stored is, of course, fat.

Calories: Enough is Enough

If you take in just as many calories as your body needs for fuel through the day, well and good. If you take in too many, your body assumes you'll find some need for them someday, and naïvely packs them away as fat. If you burn up more

106

calories than you take in, the extra amount is withdrawn from the fat on deposit.

In any plan for eating, there's an important ingredient you can't buy in any supermarket. *Exercise.* It's the one surefire way to balance the intake and output of calories so that you get the most good out of them. Physical activity enables us to get those important nutrients in food without paying the price of extra pounds.

Calories are hard to escape—a cup of instant coffee contains four calories, and a can of diet soda has just under one. Real foods, of course, are more calorie dense.

Fats and oils are the best sources of calories—a cup of butter contains 1,630! Carbohydrates, the carbon-hydrogen-oxygen molecules that abound in starches and sugars, are also good calorie sources. A cup of white sugar contains 770 calories, a cup of white flour 400.

Proteins are calorie sources, too. We sometimes think of protein-rich foods as being nearly free of calories, but this isn't true. A cup of lean ground beef has 230 calories, and so, too, does a six-ounce can of tuna fish packed in water.

Happily, many foods contain substances which aren't usable as fuel for the human machine and which, therefore, don't provide calories.

Water is an obvious example. A less obvious one is *fiber*—the various stringy, woody, gummy, spongy, and pulpy materials that give shape and substance to plants. Some animals such as cattle have complicated four-chambered stomachs that can digest fiber and derive calories from it. We can't.

Does the *number* of calories a person eats every day have anything to do with his or her risk of developing cancer?

In humans, the evidence, presented in Chapter 7, seems to point to fat, rather than calories in general, as the factor to be concerned about. We do know that the higher the per capita food intake in a country, the greater the mortality from intestinal cancers, and the lower the mortality from stomach cancer.

Another study in Hong Kong revealed that colon cancer was directly related to socioeconomic class. The most affluent group ate 3,900 calories daily and had more than *twice* the colon-cancer deaths than the poorest group, which ate only

2,700 calories daily. The richer people, of course, enjoyed a richer, fattier diet.

And in a 1975 study by Sir Richard Doll of Oxford, a comparison between total caloric intake and the cancer rates in fifty-five countries showed an association between high caloric intake and rectal cancer and leukemia in males, and breast cancer in females.

But, the NAS notes, *high-calorie diets are high in fat* and protein, particularly animal protein. To get the same calories from plant-derived foods, people would have to eat a greater volume of food, since fruits, vegetables, and whole grains contain a higher proportion of noncaloric water and fiber.

The American Cancer Society's monumental Cancer Prevention Study, conducted between 1959 and 1972, found that *serious* overweight—by forty percent or more—increased cancer mortality. Among men, overweight was linked with cancers of the colon and rectum. Among women, extra pounds meant increased cancers of the gallbladder, breast, cervix, uterus, and ovary.

It wasn't possible to ascertain the relative importance of overweight itself compared to caloric intake or other dietary factors. It can't be neatly assumed that obesity by itself will lead to cancer.

Nonetheless, the committee notes, most research has confirmed that obese people eat too many calories and, says the committee, "it is reasonable to assume that high caloric intake is a risk factor for some sites" (specific organs in the body where cancer may originate).

Was this because overweight, per se, leads to cancer, or because the fats and other calorie-dense foods that lead to overweight contain cancer-encouraging substances?

The NAS committee asked itself this question, but with the present evidence, they can't say *how* a high-calorie life-style adds to your cancer risks. The explanation might well be that those extra calories come from fat.

Proteins and Cancer

Protein foods provide not only calories but amino acids, the so-called building blocks of life. Like many clichés, this one is true. Protein foods are dismantled, during the processes of digestion, into their component parts—amino acids which the body then reassembles to make other proteins. The process is much like "cannibalizing" a car for spare parts.

What we do know about the relation between protein consumption and cancer risks is not only sparse but fuzzy. Many epidemiological studies show a strong correlation between eating a lot of protein—particularly *animal* protein—and cancers of the breast, uterus, prostate, colon, rectum, pancreas, and kidney.

That doesn't mean we should all become overnight vegetarians, since in the Western countries where these studies were done, meat, eggs, and dairy products are the favorite high-protein foods. All are great sources of *fat*, which is nobody's best friend.

High-protein diets, American style, are de facto high-fat diets, and are associated with the same patterns of cancer incidence. With our dinners of lavishly marbeled, succulent beef, and our two-eggs-over-easy breakfasts with ham, sausages, and buttered toast, a good high-protein meal inevitably turns out to be a bad high-fat meal, as well.

Fat, however, is not the only substance that piggybacks on animal protein. Meat and other major protein sources, says the NAS committee, "contain a variety of *other* nutrients and nonnutritive components[] . . . the association of protein with cancer at these sites may not be direct, but, rather, could reflect the action of another constituent concurrently present in protein-rich foods."

That, of course, does not rule out the possibility that protein or one or another of the twenty-two amino acids which string themselves together to form protein molecules might have a cancer-encouraging ability.

"The relationship of dietary protein to the carcinogenic process does not appear to be straightforward," said the committee. A little gem of scientific understatement, I think, since at two to three times the normal requirement, protein *enhances* carcinogenesis in animals, but when protein is decreased to twenty to twenty-five percent of the diet, carcinogenesis is *inhibited*!

In most animal studies, a very low protein diet suppresses carcinogenesis; in those diets, protein constitutes only five percent of what the animals eat—barely enough to sustain normal growth. No one believes that an ultra low protein diet would lower cancer risk in humans, and it would certainly undermine normal health.

Carbohydrates and Cancer

The nutritive carbohydrates, that is, the ones that provide calories, are *starches and sugars*. Very little solid research on dietary carbohydrates and cancer has been done.

Strictly speaking, fiber, too, is a carbohydrate, because of its chemical structure, but because it's not absorbed by the body, it's not considered a nutrient.

Epidemiological studies of carbohydrates and human cancer have been pathetically few and unconfirmed, and no explanations for their observations have been put forth. Some findings are interesting, but once again the NAS committee concludes that "the evidence is insufficient for firm conclusions to be drawn." In one epidemiological study, the amount of sugar people consumed was found to be linked with higher mortality from pancreatic cancer in women. In another the intake of potatoes (a good source of starch) was associated with increased mortality from cancer of the liver in both women and men. Elsewhere, a high intake of refined sugar, coupled with a low intake of starch, was linked with increased incidence of breast cancer. Both stomach cancer and cancer of the esophagus have been associated with high starch consumption.

The committee makes no recommendations about the impact of proteins or carbohydrates on cancer risks. But it makes sense not to go overboard with either of these macronutrients, for carbohydrates add calories, and protein is associated with fat.

110

12
The Mysterious Guardians

The NAS committee was clearly fascinated with what they call "inhibitors of carcinogenesis." Occurring mostly in vegetables, these are chemicals that are not, strictly speaking, necessary for nutrition. They exist in ordinary foods and, when a person eats enough of them, they can prevent carcinogenesis. There is no good, straightforward collective word for these substances, and scientists haven't much of an idea of how they might work.

It isn't even known how many of these natural inhibitors of carcinogenesis there are, whether they have all been identified, or whether some nutrients already recognized for another role in human health may double as carcinogenesis inhibitors.

No one is ready to deny that there could be compounds, present in trace amounts, that have been helping people to avoid cancer for millenia, without being identified, named, or given any credit.

"The data are of considerable interest," reports the academy committee with characteristic understatement, "even though the mechanism of inhibition is not clear."

For our purposes, it's irrelevant whether or not the scientists know what these chemicals are and how they work. These incompletely understood substances exist, they are in our foods, and a *balanced, varied, moderate* diet will provide what we need of them (so long as we don't consume too much fat, too little fiber, too much alcohol, or too many heavily salt-cured or smoked foods).

The fascinating clues to the existence of these compounds come from epidemiological studies showing that the more vegetables people eat, the fewer cancers of the gastrointestinal tract they develop. A meticulous case-control study showed that healthy controls ate more coleslaw, red cabbage, sliced tomatoes, and other vegetables than did matched patients with stomach cancer. In Japan, people who ate raw lettuce and celery had a lower risk of stomach cancer than people who didn't. Also in Japan, it was found that the risk for stomach cancer was lower among nonsmokers who ate green and yellow vegetables than for nonsmokers who did not eat them.

A case-control study of colon cancer showed that the healthy controls ate more fiber-containing foods, including cabbage; another showed that frequent consumption of cabbage, brussels sprouts, and broccoli decreased the risk for colon cancer. In a study underway, Dr. Erik Bjelke of the University of Bergen is comparing healthy cohorts of people in Minnesota and in Norway and has observed that the risk for cancers of the colon and rectum is lower among the Minnesotans who eat the most vegetables—especially cabbage.

The cruciferae (cabbage and related vegetables) are good sources of fiber and vitamin C, but so are many other vegetables. The cruciferae must contain something special.

Animal studies are the best way to search for the effects of individual constituents in the foods under scrutiny. And there are plenty of these ingredients to consider. We've already talked about the standard nutritive substances, and how they may add to or subtract from cancer risk. But there are dozens of compounds which don't belong to the familiar categories of nutrients; they're known by their biochemical family names.

Some of these families include the indoles, phenols, aromatic isothiocyanates, flavones, protease inhibitors, and something called beta-sistosterol. The category as a whole is known as the *secondary plant constituents*.

So far, animal studies show that some chemicals in this category inhibit both the initiation of the promotion phases.

Indoles, which made a splash in 1978 when Dr. Lee W. Wattenberg of the University of Minnesota reported that three of these compounds kept cancers from developing in carcinogen-treated mice, are found in the cabbage-related cruciferous vegetables, as is another class of compounds called aromatic isothiocyanates. Their exact mechanism of stopping carcinogenesis before it starts is a mystery.

Flavones are found in fruits and vegetables; some of these

112

compounds also inhibit chemically induced carcinogenesis in experimental animals. But flavones share some subtle chemical similarities to some known carcinogens. "Thus, a particular compound may have diverse effects," the committee states. "When this occurs, its overall impact is difficult to predict." Two flavones, quercetin and kaempferol, are mutagenic, according to some tests, and may—in concentrated amounts—be carcinogenic.

Another argument for the balanced, varied, moderate approach. Small doses of carcinogenic flavones, day after day after day, might cause cancerous transformation of the cells exposed to it over a couple of decades. The same compound encountered now and then could be harmless—its carcinogenic effects overriden by its anticancer action.

The moral of the story is, then, that you probably shouldn't eat the same food every single day no matter how good it is for you, or how much you like it.

Protease inhibitors stop the action of certain enzymes and also stop tumor promotion. These compounds are especially abundant in seeds. Soybeans and lima beans are excellent sources. These compounds have reduced the number of cancers developing in rats exposed to radiation, and might, the committee suggests, work together with antioxidants in inhibiting carcinogenesis.

Clues to How Cruciferae Help

A beautifully clear experiment on healthy human volunteers sums up much of the information on these mysterious guardians, and gets us away from those bewildering molecules —indoles, flavones, and protease inhibitors. The volunteers were fed large amounts of cabbage and brussels sprouts. They were also given small doses of two common drugs, phenacetin and antipyrine, which are eliminated from the body by the same biochemical pathways that rid us of many important types of carcinogens.

The researchers measured how efficiently these harmless and noncarcinogenic drugs were eliminated. "The results indicated that subjects eating diets rich in the vegetables metabolized both drugs more rapidly than did subjects on a control diet," the NSA committee reports.

The cruciferae-rich diet made those built-in clean-up systems work more efficiently, and the commonsense inference is that if cruciferae enable us to get rid of the harmless compounds better, they will probably do the same for chemicals in related compounds that can cause cancer.

(No ethical experimenter would dream of performing the experiment that would clinch the argument perfectly. That would be to feed people *known* carcinogens and see whether a cabbage-and-brussels sprouts diet would make them detoxify these compounds faster than a control diet.)

Note that the *whole*, garden-variety vegetable is used to make this experimental point. Except for normal preparation and cooking, nothing was done to the food, and no attempt was made to concentrate or manipulate it. There were no sprout extracts, no indole capsules, no *eau de chou*.

In the wake of this report, nimble manufacturers will start advertising all kinds of untested, unproved products of this nature, promising wondrous cancer protection.

Don't buy them. Flavone pills and other "natural" supplements may do much more harm than good, particularly if you take them every day. Nobody really knows enough about them to justify advising healthy people to take in large amounts of these compounds. We know they are powerful—we don't know the possible harm that overdosing might do.

Instead, I urge you to make friends with the produce manager at your supermarket, or the nice family who runs the vegetable store, and start getting better acquainted with the cabbages, and the brussels sprouts, the cauliflower and the bok choy, the broccoli, the kale, the Napa cabbage, the kohlrabi, and the rest of the wonderful vegetables listed on page 164.

13
Additives and Contaminants

People are probably less worried about the subtle role of zinc, or the hazards of old-fashioned preserving methods, than they are about newfangled chemicals with multisyllabic names that have entered our food supply since our grandparents' day. No-calorie sweeteners, antioxidants, and all kinds of "additives" are put in to enhance the flavor, color, or shelf life of our foods. We're assured that they are safe, but these days we're skeptical.

And if a person is concerned about cancer risk, is it safe to eat products containing those ingredients with difficult chemical names which often outnumber familiar substances like sugar and flour on the label?

Additives: Natural and Not

Some of the nonfood ingredients we find in our food are, indeed, wholly man-made and aren't found anywhere in nature. BHA, the antioxidant, is one. Ethylenediamine tetraacetic acid (EDTA), used to neutralize metallic impurities that would otherwise discolor food and spoil it, is another.

Some additives, like sugar (from plants such as sugar cane, sugar beets, or corn), are derived from natural sources. Monosodium glutamate, the flavor amplifier, is another example that you may not know about. Despite its moniker, it isn't the brainchild of a mad organic chemist. It originates in corn.

Some additives are cheap but identical copies of natural compounds—sodium propionate, a widely used preservative, was first discovered in cheese. It prevents mold from growing on food.

Nearly 3,000 substances are knowingly added to foods

during processing in the United States, and an estimated 12,000 wander into our food during production, processing, or packaging.

In her excellent *Nutrition Book* (Bantam Books), Jane E. Brody estimates that the average adult American consumes about 150 pounds of "additives" every year. Of that total, 95 pounds is sugar; 33 pounds come from other sweeteners like corn syrup, dextrose, and such; and 15 pounds of the additive total is salt. In addition, common additives like pepper, yeast, vinegar, mustard, and MSG contribute 9 pounds a year.

The rest—about a pound—comes from another 2,600 additives. We consume about half of them in amounts of less than 0.5 milligrams a year.

The Delaney Clause

In 1958, Congress took official cognizance of the possibility that some food additives might be carcinogenic, and in amending the Food, Drug, and Cosmetic Act of 1938, put in the famed Delaney Clause, sometimes called the Delaney Amendment.

This much-praised, much-criticized piece of legislation decrees that no additive can be used in food if it causes cancer in either people or animals, or is found to cause cancer "in tests appropriate for the evaluation of the safety of food additives." Under the Delaney Clause, the Food and Drug Administration has banned three food-coloring agents, a flavoring used in aperitif wines, and safrole, a derivative of the sassafras root formerly used to flavor root beer and sarsaparilla. (But sassafras root still appears in some herbal teas available at health food stores!)

As has happened when political decisions are made before the relevant scientific evidence has been gathered and weighed, the well-intentioned Delaney Clause turns out to be scientifically naïve, and easily torpedoed politically.

Food additives are tested one by one for carcinogenicity, but that doesn't address the practical question: How do they interact with each other, in our varied American diet? Can cocarcinogens cause cancers that neither compound could cause alone? Even though the combination punch of initiation and promotion is crucial in the process of carcinogenesis, the interaction of additives hasn't been looked at yet.

Nor has anyone determined how protective substances like vitamin C, beta-carotene, or secondary plant constituents could inhibit a compound's carcinogenic effect in the test situation. The additives that people consume constitute a small fraction of the food intake, and many important foods we love (or could easily learn to love) are formidable defenders against cancer. A balanced, varied, moderate diet may simply overwhelm weak carcinogens in the amounts people actually eat.

But, under the Delaney Clause, *any compound that causes cancer in laboratory animals is disallowed*.

That's a big inconvenience for food producers sometimes, such as when a popular additive like red dye no. 4 was banned. They put up a predictable fight when a useful, commercially popular, and, in their honest opinion, harmless ingredient had to go. There are, however, plenty of other food colors around.

Things get politically hairy when, under the Delaney Clause, the FDA is compelled to ban a profitable substance for which no good substitute exists. It's even more of a Capitol Hill nightmare when the public perceives that the compound under fire has benefits for them—real or imagined. This was what happened with saccharin.

The coal-tar derivative, beloved of diet-soda addicts, weight watchers, and diabetics, has been used as a calorie-free sweetener since 1907. Unlike most additives, saccharin has a track record in human use long enough for any marked carcinogenic effect to have revealed itself. In large groups of people in both the United States and Great Britain, however, epidemiologists have found no such trend.

No one can say whether that means it's completely safe. *Weak* carcinogens don't have much numerical impact either in human epidemiology or in animal experiments. Remember that fewer mice are needed to detect a powerful effect than are required to study a weak carcinogen that affects only a small percentage of the animals.

Though some case-control studies showed that *men* (not women) who used artificial sweeteners had an elevated risk of bladder cancer, later, larger studies haven't confirmed it.

The NAS committee quoted the International Agency for Research on Cancer's 1980 conclusion that "although a small increase in the risk of urinary bladder cancer in the general population or a larger increase in some individuals consuming very high doses of saccharin cannot be excluded, the epidemiological data provide no clear evidence that saccharin alone, or in combination with cyclamates, causes urinary bladder cancer." (Cyclamates are other calorie-free artificial sweeteners, no longer used in the U.S. because it's agreed they *do* pose a cancer risk.)

Saccharin, at high doses, promotes urinary cancer in male rats and can act as a promoter, cooperating with known carcinogens, in the bladders of rats of both sexes. Evidence that saccharin is carcinogenic in *mice*, however, is limited. Mutagenicity studies such as the Ames test indicate that saccharin is weakly mutagenic.

The consensus is that saccharin itself is not much of a carcinogen when acting alone, but when combined with promoters, it *may* carry some risk.

Unconvinced either way by the available evidence, the NAS committee said nothing specific about saccharin.

And it appears we no longer have to be concerned about diethylstilbestrol (DES) in our food. The hormone helps cattle grow faster, and was a great favorite with the meat industry. Minute amounts of DES residues remained in the meat after the animals were slaughtered, and were presumably eaten by people. These scant amounts of DES were never associated with cancer in humans, but DES was given in much larger doses to pregnant women to prevent miscarriage, and the children of some of these women developed genital cancers in adolescence. DES was banned in 1972, against stiff resistance by the meat industry. Even after the ban, some producers continued to use the hormone illegally for several years, but it's been abandoned.

As for the rest of the additives that comprise that one pound total in the yearly diet of an American, only small numbers have been tested, and of these, only a relative few were studied using methods that met the committee's standards.

"There is no evidence suggesting that the increasing use of food additives has contributed significantly to the overall risk of cancer for humans," the committee concludes, hastening to add that the lack of evidence doesn't guarantee that all is hunky-dory in the wonderful world of additives.

Additives may have a real, albeit invisible, drop-in-the-bucket effect. It may be that additives may cause a small increase in cancer incidence which is undetectable against the background of common cancers caused by cigarette smoking and too much fat in the diet.

It may be that they haven't had time to cause enough cancers for epidemiologists to find them, because synthetic food additives didn't enter common use in a big way until comparatively recently.

Or it may be that, like saccharin, most food additives are such ineffective carcinogens, if they're carcinogenic at all, and present in such minute amounts, that they aren't adding anything to anybody's risk of cancer.

An Additive on Our Side

And at least one additive seems to be wearing a good-guy white hat. BHA (butylated hydroxyanisole) is widely used to prevent spoilage—most of us eat a little of it every day. Study after study in animals shows that BHA has real cancer-inhibiting powers. When administered before and during exposure to carcinogens, BHA acts as a blocking agent, and it inhibits the second, promoting step of carcinogenesis. Furthermore, it stymies the DNA-damaging effects of mutagens.

Interestingly, BHA, a synthetic chemical, is structurally similar to some of the known natural inhibitors of carcinogenesis discussed in Chapter 12. It belongs to the chemical family known as the *phenols*.

At most, we eat only a few milligrams of BHA each day, from various processed foods. This is far, far less, per pound of body weight, than the amount of this phenol given to laboratory mice in carcinogenesis-blocking experiments. Perhaps we don't ingest enough BHA to do us any good against cancer. On the other hand, the laboratory animals received massive doses of chemical carcinogens in those experiments. So it's possible that even the minute amounts of BHA we eat every day are enough to act against some of the carcinogens in our lives.

It's an open question. The committee warns, "No conclusions can be drawn at this time as to whether inhibitory effects of BHA occur at the low concentrations of carcinogens to which humans are generally exposed."

Contaminants

Your food contains some substances that don't belong there at all. But the amounts are so low that they pose no cancer threat, so far as is known.

Occasionally, vinyl chloride and acrylonitrile, both used in food packaging, get into foods in infinitesimal amounts. Both these compounds are carcinogenic in animals, and vinyl chloride is a potent human carcinogen (one of the few that nobody argues about). But there is no indication that anyone gets cancer from the very small amounts that occasionally drift into foods by accident. Our bodies probably detoxify and eliminate these tiny doses effectively.

Some *pesticides*, notably kepone, toxaphene, hexachlorobenzene, and perhaps heptachlor, can enter food and drinking water and, because they're carcinogenic to animals, the levels of these compounds are monitored clearly by the FDA's Market Basket Survey of everyday foods. Fortunately, the levels are consistently very low, and the NAS committee says, "the amounts present in the average U.S. diet do not make a major contribution to the overall risk of cancer for humans."

Polychlorinated biphenyls, or PCB's, are industrial chemicals commonly used for the past fifty years, some of which are mutagenic in the Ames test and carcinogenic in some laboratory animals. PCB's have a nasty way of getting into the food chain and staying there, going from soil or water into plants, then moving into the tissues of animals and fish that eat the plants, and staying stubbornly in the humans who eventually eat PCB-containing foods.

These compounds, like the pesticides, are carefully monitored in the FDA Market Basket Survey, and occur in amounts way below the FDA's tolerance levels.

Polybrominated biphenyls (PBB's) are close relatives of PCB's and similarly persist in the environment, accumulating in human fat. No epidemiological data show any impact of PBB's on cancer risk or general human health, but PBB's *can* produce cancers in laboratory animals.

Polycyclic aromatic hydrocarbons (PAH's) in the environment number more than one hundred. Workers exposed occupationally to these compounds have an increased incidence of skin and lung cancers. One of the PAH's—benzo (a) pyrene—is such an efficient carcinogen that a *single dose* of the stuff can cause stomach cancer in mice.

The carcinogenicity of PAH's extends along the spectrum from potent to very weak. As we've seen, this family of compounds is under close scrutiny, most notably by Dr. Sugimura and his Japanese colleagues, since PAH's exist in so many foods besides the grilled meat and fish where they first came to the attention of cancer scientists.

There are PAH's in fresh and smoked meats and fish, leafy and root vegetables, oils, grains, fruits, seafoods, whiskeys, foods that have been cooked at high temperatures, even in coffee beans dried with hot air!

The NAS committee views all these molecules with caution. "There is no epidemiological evidence to suggest that these compounds individually make a major contribution to the risk of human cancer," they say.

However, they continue, we can't rule out the possibility that these substances act synergistically, helping each other out and creating a greater risk than the contaminants present individually.

14
Balanced, Varied, and Moderate

As Dr. Grobstein, Dr. Mertz, and many other members of the committee emphasize, the scientific evidence about diet and cancer points to a need for a balanced, varied, moderate diet. How can we achieve this goal?

Balance

If our stomachs could hold all the food we wanted to eat, and if calories didn't count, it would be easy to achieve optimum nutrition.

But getting what we need from food without taking in too many calories is like a problem in economics.

Think of the ideal daily allowance of calories as *income*—your "calorie salary." Think of your nutritional needs—protein, fatty acids, fiber, vitamins, minerals, trace elements, cancer-preventing agents, and other life-sustaining substances—as financial obligations. We have to balance our nutritional books—calories weighed against nutrients.

Since virtually everything you eat contains some energy value, you have to "spend" calories to get from your food the nutrients you need, the same way that your everyday necessities cost you money. If you blow your paycheck on a trip to Bermuda, you won't have enough in the bank to cover your rent. If your day's activities require 2,000 calories, you could spend them all on ten Hershey bars with almonds, but that would leave you starved for protein, fiber, and micronutrients. Eating other foods in order to get those important nutrients means taking in more calories, over and above the 2,000 you burn up. The excess is stored as fat.

Nutritionists say that a person has to take in a minimum of

,600 calories to obtain a day's worth of nutrients. The secret of good nutritional management, like good financial management, is to hold out for good value.

Butter, for example, is a source of vitamin A. A cup of butter contains 150 retinol equivalents—the units of measure. But it also contains 184 grams of fat and 1,630 calories! On the other hand, a cup of fresh cooked carrots contains more than twice as much beta-carotene, just a smidgin of fat, and only 50 calories. As a vitamin A source, butter is not much of a bargain, but carrots are.

If you try to figure out how to pay for all the nutrients you need with your daily calorie allowance, you'll get bogged down in a tangle of supply-side economics which would require an accountant as well as a nutrition scientist to straighten out.

Fortunately, we don't have to plan each day's food separately. "The body has sufficient reserves to make it possible to think in terms of a balanced *weekly* diet," says USDA's Dr. Walter Mertz. "What matters is your nutritional total for the week, not what you eat in a single day."

That's nice for two reasons. One is that it spares us a lot of tedious arithmetic at the dinner table and in the kitchen. The other is that we can *vary* the way we spend our calorie salary from day to day. Like "saving up" for a special purchase by walking instead of taking buses, or making up for a financial binge by economizing afterward, you can compensate for a calorie splurge by eating lightly before a big party, or emphasizing fruits and vegetables for a day or so after a weekend of indulgence.

A healthy adult can get away with a *day* of dietary extremism, providing his or her overall diet is balanced, varied, and moderate. One day of a strict vegeterian regime won't hurt you, nor will one day of a liquid diet food, or even an oddball fad diet or a total fast—IF, during the rest of your week, you plan your eating to account for your nutritional requirements.

One day of junk food or gourmet luxury will neither wreck your health, ruin your figure, nor increase your risk of cancer, *so long as you make up for your excesses*. There are lots of ways. When you know that dinner will be special, anticipate it with a light breakfast and a lunch hour spent walking or shopping instead of eating. Or you can eat smaller portions of everything for a couple of days before a luxurious meal.

Some splurges, of course, can't be planned for. I strive to compensate for unexpected feasts *immediately*, while the memory is still fresh. Fruit and tea for breakfast the next day, a salad lunch, a lean dinner. You could, alternatively, make across-the-board calorie cutbacks for a few days, by eating very dainty portions of all your foods, eliminating all cooking oils and fats, and cutting way down on carbohydrates, but some of us prefer to do our compensating quickly. I once knew a woman who loved to eat and entertained lavishly every weekend. Every Monday she ate nothing but apples, and drank black coffee, and water. She'd been compensating in that extremist fashion for years and it seemed to have done her no harm.

"If you feast one day, you can balance things out the next," says Dr. Mertz.

Variety

Most people enjoy variety in their meals. Perhaps nature recognizes that if you eat the same food every day, you will miss out on important nutrients, while subjecting yourself to repeated doses of compounds that may cause harm.

When you suddenly go "off your feed," as my grandmother used to put it, when you crave new tastes and textures and a change from your usual fare, your body may be telling you something important. Variety isn't just the spice of life, it may even *save* your life from cancer.

The appealing principle of variety in eating makes it much easier to follow the other principles of balance and moderation, and helps make up for the effort and discipline we need in order to develop better eating habits.

The U.S. Department of Agriculture's booklet *Nutrition and Your Health: Dietary Guidelines for Americans* sets forth in more specific terms the principles of balance, variety, and moderation implicit in the NAS committee report.

The USDA says, "You should eat a variety of foods to assure an adequate diet. The greater the variety, the less likely you are to develop either a deficiency or an excess of any single nutrient. Variety also reduces your likelihood of

124

being exposed to excessive amounts of contaminants in any single food item.''

There's a simple way to arrive at variety, and balance, too. Just remember the four major food groups and choose some foods, each day, from each group.

- Fruits and vegetables (including starchy vegetables and legumes)
- Whole-grain and enriched breads, cereals, and grain products
- Milk, cheese, and yogurt
- Meats, fish, poultry, eggs

Variety means a variety of cooking styles, not just a variety of foods. When I accepted the fact that eating forty percent of my calories in the form of fat was making me a candidate for cancer, I started looking for alternatives to cooking in fat. Since low-fat cuisines from the Orient are associated with lower incidence of breast and colon cancers, I decided to explore the wonderful world of the wok.

This bowl-shaped iron cooking pot focuses the heat so that food can be prepared deliciously with very little cooking oil. You can cook a vast mound of fresh vegetables quickly (saving on cooking fuel) and in just a few teaspoons of oil. More recent developments in low-fat cooking are the non-stick frying pan and griddles, and the spray-on lubricants which keep food from sticking or burning in ordinary cookware. Over a year's time, they can help you avoid a considerable amount of the fats and oils used not to make food taste better but just to facilitate cooking.

If, in the course of balancing out your week's food, you want to include a meatless day to compensate for a high-fat indulgence, a bigger serving of one of the whole grains, nicely dressed up with mushrooms and onions, can be the centerpiece for a vegetarian dinner. They are virtually fat free and a splendid source of the pentosan fraction of fiber, besides being loaded with nutrients.

You see how variety can not only make sensible eating a pleasure instead of a sacrifice, it can also keep boredom away from the dinner table. Variety as a dietary principle also means that you can eat things that aren't very good for you, once in a while. You can even enjoy Icelandic salted fish, if that's your pleasure, as a now-and-then treat, so long as you continue adventuring with a variety of other kinds of foods in the meantime.

Moderation

Balance and variety in your diet make moderation easy, and healthy nutrition a matter of pleasure and excitement rather than willpower.

To get all the other nutrients you need, and still stay within your calorie allowance, some adjustments in the amount of high-fat dairy products and some meats will probably be in order. Don't worry—with the increased amount of filling vegetables and whole grains a balanced diet will entail, you won't go hungry.

If you expand your range of choices to include new and interesting recipes and a more adventuresome repertoire of choices, your more moderate diet will feel like an adventure, instead of a sacrifice. For example, where is it decreed that meat must be the main dish at your evening meal? Your meat, exotically prepared as an hors d'oeuvre or finger food to enjoy with your predinner drink, can serve as a prelude to a meal of hearty soup, salad, and whole-grain bread.

When you expand your ideas of what a meal should or should not be, and start cooking in more adventurous and creative ways, moderation in fat and calories comes easily. You won't want to eliminate fat entirely but you may find, as I have, that with the fat-sparing tricks mentioned above, and with menus that provide good protein from low-fat sources like fish, poultry, or lean red meat, a day can pass without your eating much fat at all. When your food is exciting and satisfying in its own right, you won't miss the fat.

That's lovely, because we want to indulge in blatantly rich foods now and then. In March, when the first fresh asparagus appears, I love to make a whole lunch or dinner out of thick, carefully peeled spears with classic butter-and-egg hollandaise sauce. That indulgence uses up the butter for about three days, and two of my three weekly egg yolks in one splendid swoop. But with some low-fat days in the bank, so to speak, I can afford it.

This principle holds true for all the substances associated

126

with increased cancer risk—foods preserved by heavy smoking or salting; alcohol; fats—and the welter of food additives that haven't been tested for carcinogenicity. You can enjoy these suspect foods safely now and then, if you've learned to build your *regular* diet around foods that pose no cancer threat.

I've already discussed some ways in which a balanced and varied diet will help bring your daily fat intake down toward the moderate thirty percent level. Moderating alcohol consumption is a touchy matter—nobody who enjoys a drink wants to be told to drink less.

Complicating the issue further is the medical evidence that those who abstain from alcohol completely have a greater risk of high blood pressure and heart trouble. Must we choose among a risk of oral, esophageal, and liver cancers and a risk of heart attack?

No. A drink or two per day is fine. If you have something to eat along with your evening highball, or drink your wine with your dinner, so much the better. The food may protect the tissues exposed to the alcohol. And, because you're striving to keep your calorie budget balanced, there will be some evenings when you'll want to spend the calories (100 per glass of beer, the equivalent of 10 teaspoons of sugar) on something else (4 tablespoons of sour cream on your chili). Skipping your nightly drink now and then breaks the sequence of cancer-promoting events that even a light alcohol intake may cause.

Special occasions seem to call for more than a glass of white wine. So long as you don't extend the definition of special occasion to include every weekend (let alone every night), occasional excesses aren't likely to raise your cancer risk.

If you can't live comfortably within these moderate limits, then alcohol may pose threats to your health and happiness more immediate than the possibility of cancer twenty years from now.

If you are a heavy drinker and a smoker, as well, your chances of developing cancer are increased far beyond the separate risks involved in either smoking or drinking.

Two Practical Plans

If the scientific evidence has convinced you that what you eat affects your chances of developing cancer, and if you are seriously interested in making the NAS committee's guidelines work for you, you can choose between two very different approaches to a balanced, varied, moderate diet.

One is to switch over completely to a well-thought-out plan that embodies all the lessons of the NAS report: less fat; more fiber; greater emphasis on fruits, vegetables, and whole grains; and a limited intake of alcohol and heavily salted foods. Such "prudent" diets have been devised by a number of authorities. By following them, you can be fairly certain you're getting all your necessary nutrients without exceeding the proper number of calories.

The second approach is to stay with your present eating patterns while introducing new habits, modifying recipes, trying out new menus, and doing things a bit differently in the kitchen and on your shopping rounds. Since the dietary changes recommended by the NAS committee are not really radical departures from the way most Americans eat, modest alterations here and there can add up to an overall diet in keeping with the guidelines, and even small changes will be better than none at all. It's not an all-or-nothing matter.

The route you take to lowering your cancer risks through dietary change is really up to you. Some people enjoy totally new beginnings, following a clear plan. Others prefer a more informal and experimental style.

This book offers you *both*. Chapter 18 presents a comprehensive approach to good nutrition, based on Ideas for Better Eating, a program created by the Human Nutrition Information Service at the U.S. Department of Agriculture. It's based on an ingenious and very simple system of "trade-offs," rather than calorie-counting, which enables you to vary your food choices comfortably while maintaining good nutrition and staying within your daily calorie limit. It's a very livable diet, easily adapted to family life where different people require different amounts of calories.

With a few minor modifications—such as focusing explicitly on cruciferous vegetables, instead of including them among all the other green and leafy things—the Everyday Food Plans in this book are based directly on USDA information. Except where other agencies and institutions are credited, the material in this section is all based on the USDA nutritionists' commonsense approach.

For people who for one reason or another don't want to commit themselves to any specific dietary regime, even one as comfortable as the USDA's, the next two chapters provide plenty of practical suggestions and assistance in reshaping your attitudes toward food. If you start gradually with the ideas that seem most congenial to you, then add others as time goes on, you will introduce some significant reforms in your overall diet, without expending a great deal of effort or willpower.

Whichever your preference, I urge you to read both the chapter on Working Toward an Anticancer Life-style (Chapter 15) and the Everyday Food Plans (Chapter 18). Whichever course you decide to take, you will find explanation of the other helpful. The basic principles are the same, and the recipes in Chapter 19 can be used in either case.

15
Working Toward an Anticancer Life-style

My first dietary change came from the realization that much of the fat in my diet came from *cheese*. Cheese is delicious, and it's wonderful *food*. An ounce of Monterey Jack, my favorite, contains 15 grams of protein. Alas, one ounce also has 8 grams of fat! A total of 100 calories!

Before I got serious about reducing my cancer risks, I always kept a goodly hunk of cheese in the refrigerator, so I could have a nibble whenever I felt the need. I harbored the illusion that my cheesy snacking didn't *count*. After learning how much fat was concealed in the Fontina, I realized I'd better eat less.

I reduced my cheese intake with a trick so simple I'm almost embarrassed to describe it. I bought a cheese scraper—an implement that looks something like a pancake turner, with a sharp edge in the middle. The scraper—otherwise known as a cheese plane—is designed so you *can't* cut a piece thicker than a piece of paper. When you draw it across the face of a piece of cheese, you get a thin, elegant curl, not a gross chunk. Now I habitually use the scraper instead of a knife and find that the pound of cheese that I used to go through in a couple of days now lasts a week.

Sneaking Up on a Low-Fat Life

Reducing the size of your portions is a sound and easy way to cut down on fat. The simple expedient of making one more hamburger from a pound of ground meat can make a significant difference: instead of four quarter-pounders, make five patties of about three ounces each. If that gives you an extra, wrap it in plastic and freeze it.

Here are a few of my favorite little tricks for cutting out a little fat here and there. Even if you follow all of them, you can't achieve the cancer-protective effect you'd obtain if you made a serious effort to get your fat below thirty percent of your calories. But you will do yourself *some* good, while developing some low-fat habits that will make further reductions easier.

- Trim visible fat from your meat on your dinner plate. Such a simple, practical step, and perhaps the most important single action you can take to reduce your dietary fat. Set your table with steak knives—even when you're not eating steak—as a reminder to cut the fat away.
- Buy a nonstick frying pan. You'd be surprised how much fat and oil you use not so much for flavor as to avoid burning fried foods and messing up the pan.
- Buy a can of Pam, the spray-on lubricant for your conventional cooking pots and pans, and keep it near the stove so you'll remember to use it. Spraying the inside of a cake pan or a casserole will not only save you a few fat-calories (not many, but they add up over a period of time) but will remind you of your reduced-fat goals.
- When starting a stew or a sauce, cook the onions, peppers, garlic, etc., in ½ cup of white wine instead of butter or oil. As the wine evaporates, the vegetables cook and soften, so that you can even brown them as the pan dries, if you stir carefully to prevent burning.
- Buy strongly flavored oils—like Greek olive oil and sesame-seed oil—and use a few drops for flavoring, instead of using larger quantities of milder-flavored oils. In a salad dressing calling for two tablespoonfuls of olive oil, for instance, I use a teaspoonful of the good green Greek kind, and make up the rest of the volume with water.
- Buy a bottle of Liquid Smoke (E. H. Wright Co., P.O. Drawer 899, Brentwood, Tennessee 37027) and use it instead of bacon or ham when you want a smoky taste.
- Stop spreading butter or margarine on your bread. If it's decent bread (some good recipes follow), you don't need fatty spreads. If you must have something on your morn-

ing toast or muffins, use low-fat cottage cheese, or even a bit of honey or jam. Sure, these contain calories from sugar, but they don't carry the cancer danger that goes with fat calories. Save your butter allotment for some better use, where nothing else will do, and use margarine as a last-resort spread.

- The dairy industry has come up with all kinds of ingenious low-fat versions of favorite foods. *Use them!* Low-fat (1 or 2 percent fat) milk is a godsend, and if you haven't tried it, I urge you to start now. Many people dislike skim milk because it can seem thin and watery compared to whole milk. Low-fat milk starts as skim, but contains extra milk solids for body and flavor. It's sold under cutesy names like Brisk and Bouncy, or Lite 'n Lively.

- Use imitation cream cheese (4 grams of fat and 50 calories per ounce) or Neufchatel (6 grams of fat and 70 calories) instead of cream cheese (10 grams of fat, 100 calories). As spreads and as ingredients in cooking, they're indistinguishable from the old-fashioned kind.

- Get rid of excess fat before you cook. One ounce of fat on a pork roast equals 25 grams of fat and over 230 fat calories. Meat is easier to trim when it's cold and the fat is clearly visible.

- Before you cook chicken, peel the skin away. That's where a lot of the fat is concentrated. Yes, you can take the skin from a chicken before you roast it whole—it comes off like a sweater from a slightly reluctant three-year-old. With the large cavity facing you, work your fingers between the skin and the breast meat to loosen it, then pull the skin toward the neck of the bird. Grasp the skin at the point where the legs meet the body, and slip down each leg, turning the skin inside out. You can grip it more securely if you grasp the skin with a piece of dry paper towel. Cook the skinned bird in a covered pan to keep it from drying out; sprinkle with a little paprika and let it brown, uncovered, for the last few minutes of cooking.

- Chicken wings make fine appetizers or finger food, however, the skin is full of fat and is difficult to remove from wings when they're raw. But if you simmer them in water for eight or ten minutes, the cooked skin slips right off. You can complete the cooking of the meaty parts in many delectable ways—barbecued, curried, with soy sauce and fresh ginger . . .

Reducing fat is, of course, the most important step you can take to reduce your dietary risks of cancer, but as the guidelines imply, the lowering of fat should be accomplished by an increase in the protective vegetables and fruits and whole grains.

Stepping Up the Fiber

Again, there are small, painless ways to improve your diet's anticancer effects.

- Make it a project to discover new vegetables. In recent years, the variety and fascination of the supermarket produce departments have absolutely bloomed. You've surely noticed the purple cauliflower, the wealth of new exotic-looking squashes. Every week there seems to be a new variety of lettuce or greens. Have you tried even half of these newcomers? Don't stick with the tried-and-true vegetables you've been eating all your life; experiment with the new ones and bring some added variety to your table.
- Start eating those bits of fresh garniture that restaurants and hostesses add to your plate as decorations—the parsley, the fresh radish, the carrot curl. No, the tiny amount of fiber and vitamins you add to your daily food intake will not make a great deal of difference to your biochemical balance—but you'll be raising your consciousness, so to speak, about the need for fresh things. Even if you aren't a salad eater, you can manage to munch down that little scrap of chicory or slice of tomato that graces your hamburger platter.
- Choose whole-grain bread, crackers, and baked goods. Specify whole wheat when ordering a sandwich; pass up the saltines for whole-wheat crackers; order a bran muffin instead of an English. Of all the changes I've made in my diet, this has been the easiest. The difference in flavor between commercial whole-wheat bread and the

white "enriched" kind is scarcely noticeable, and it isn't hard to get used to the darker bread. After that, it's a simple and delicious step to real, hearty, whole-grain homemade bread. But you can start small, with Scandinavian flatbreads or Ry-Krisp instead of ordinary crackers. And certainly, if you are serving a sumptuous, fatty cheese, or a meaty appetizer like cocktail frankfurters, they should be accompanied by a fiber-rich bread or cracker.

- Use carrots and other fresh, raw vegetables as foils for dips and spreads. The French call them *crudités,* and they make a pretty, low-calorie, festive display when served with your predinner drink or with soup. Spread Neufchatel cheese (softened with yogurt and spiced with chives, herbs, chopped hot peppers) on slices of cucumber, green peppers, and zucchini. And who says you have to use greasy potato chips to scoop up a dip? Use broccoli flowerets, carrot sticks, summer squash. You don't need a cracker to carry a piece of cheese—use a broad slice of celery, a radish, a firm square cut from a cabbage leaf.
- Make a point of eating *something* that's raw and fresh with each meal—a glass of orange juice or a slice of melon with breakfast. Coleslaw or sliced tomatoes with lunch. A green salad with dinner. Don't think in terms of abstaining or depriving yourself—recognize that you are adding satisfying, health-enhancing foods to your everyday diet.

Increasing Beta-carotene

- Make friends with carrots. These cheap, humble vegetables look so bright and cheerful when they're scrubbed clean and cut into strips. Children love carrot sticks—keep them in a jar or plastic container of water in the refrigerator to keep them crisp for snacking.
- Mash carrots as you would potatoes; moisten with low-fat milk or lemon juice. Season with grated orange or orange juice concentrate; with lemon juice and fresh dill; with cinnamon, nutmeg, and a touch of honey. Serve whole boiled carrots in a sauce of yogurt and curry powder with grated onion.

134

- Add grated carrots to ground meat for meat loaf, stuffed vegetables, hamburgers—a good way to stretch meat economically without adding the starch of bread crumbs.
- Children are especially fascinated with carrots grated in the rotary, hand-held French grater called a Mouli. This makes a very fine, curly mass of shreds which look marvelous on top of a salad or as a garnish for cooked vegetables of any kind. You can add Mouli-shredded carrots to cookies and desserts that call for coconut—the flavor isn't the same but the texture is pretty close, and carrots don't contain the hard saturated fat that's present in coconut. Try shredded carrots in anything involving chocolate—brownies, chocolate-chip cookies, and so forth.

Getting More of the Guardians

- Strive to eat a serving of at least one cruciferous vegetable every day. There are so many different kinds, you can go for a couple of weeks without repeating. If you really don't like the cabbagy taste, don't serve them as vegetables. Add chopped cabbage to soups and stews, use chopped kale in stuffings or add it to meat loaf. When cooked together with onions in savory dishes, cruciferae lose their assertiveness, and when added raw to salads, cabbage at least doesn't have much taste at all. On the other hand, if you're a real cabbage-lover, you'll strengthen its flavor if you add a little prepared mustard.
- Start enjoying the seasonal fruits. The parade of fresh fruits that arrives with each season gives us a wonderful opportunity to build a varied, interesting diet. As the peaches pass their prime, you can look forward to the apples and the grapefruit. If you stay in a rut, eating the same fruit the year round, as you can if your supermarket is well supplied, you may be missing out on some important micronutrient not present in your customary apple a day.

Now there are substances that *do* add to our cancer risk. Fat, of course, is the biggest threat to Americans, but there are others.

Alcohol, nitrites, nitrates, and nitrosamines, to name a few. Some of the mutagens present in foods cooked at high temperatures. Some of the additives and contaminants in processed foods. And nature has its own powerful carcinogens: aflatoxin, the product of a mold that may grow on improperly stored peanuts, corn, or other grains; some compounds called hydrazines, present in wild mushrooms, are carcinogenic to mice; wild bracken fern, a delicacy in Japan, contains carcinogens.

You probably don't indulge often in bracken-fern brunches, but you may be worried about the other items. Should you swear them all off forever, or feel guilty when you offer them to your family or your guests?

Hardly. People have been enjoying these foods for centuries, but we should remember the lessons from the laboratory animals—that cancer is the end result of a lengthy process of initiation and promotion.

By *varying* our diet, experimenting with different foods, deliberately not eating the same old thing every day, we interrupt the carcinogenic scenario. Promotion must be repeated for cancer to occur.

Eating a charcoal-broiled burger every weekday for lunch throughout your working life could be risky. Eating one now and then probably won't hurt you, since the epithelial cells of the gastrointestinal lining have a chance to return to normal between encounters with promoters.

Here are three easy ways to stop repeating doses of possible promoters:

- Consider alternatives to saccharin-sweetened diet sodas and alcoholic drinks which may add to your cancer risk. The simplest and cheapest is plain water. True, in some parts of the country minute amounts of suspect chemicals may appear in drinking water, but the committee found no evidence of any impact on cancer risk. If you're concerned, or if tap water doesn't appeal to you, start discovering bottled waters—from good old seltzer and club soda to the imported kinds, both sparkling and still. They all have slightly different personalities, many contain important trace minerals, and not one has a single calorie!

  You can also buy a device which makes sparkling water cheaply from tap water and an inexpensive carbon-dioxide cartridge. For flavor, add a twist of lemon or lime or a dash of vanilla or bitters. A friend of mine who turned toward soda water when he stopped drinking alcohol adds a teaspoonful of Tabasco sauce to each glass of sparkling water. I haven't tried that one yet.

- Save your backyard grill for special summer evenings— don't make it a cookout every night. Use a few drops of Liquid Smoke to impart a smoky flavor to meats cooked at moderate temperatures on the stove.

  Or if you want to keep your kitchen cool, use the outdoor grill or hibachi in new ways. Try cooking foods inside little packages of aluminum foil. Put a piece of chicken on a square of foil, douse it with soy sauce or white wine, add some onion slices and seasonings, and wrap it like an air-tight parcel to cook on the grill. Package any kind of fish with a slice of lemon, tomato, and onion, topped with a bay leaf, and cook the same way.

- When you *do* have a traditional backyard barbecue, be lavish with the protective foods: coleslaw, raw tomatoes, carrot sticks, spinach salad, and fresh fruits.

16
Planning Your Food Strategy

The balanced, varied, moderate meals you should strive for, most days, require much less conscious planning than you might think because these three dietary virtues really reinforce each other. Naturally, you'll want to keep within your calorie limit—while you take in enough fiber, protein, and micronutrients—and keep your fat intake low, but you needn't drive yourself crazy with bookkeeping. It's a matter of changing your attitudes, following a few simple rules, and staying aware of what you eat from day to day.

The principles to bear in mind:

1) Have some meat, poultry, or fish every day. Trim away the visible fat before cooking, and stick to the leaner cuts of meat.
2) Use low-fat dairy products routinely. Recognize the hidden fats in your foods—such as sauces, mixes, "convenience foods," canned and frozen main dishes, salad dressings, baked goods—using a good guide like *The Brand-Name Nutrition Counter*.
3) Allow yourself *three or four egg yolks each week*—and as many egg whites as you like.
4) Try to arrange your food so that as nearly as possible, one-third of your daily fat comes from butter, eggs, dairy products, or meat (the saturated sources); one-third from peanut, sesame, or olive oil (monounsaturated); one-third from corn oil and other polyunsaturated sources. You can switch the proportions around from day to day so long as you don't exceed the one-third/one-third/one-third ratio over a week's time.

5) You need fruits and vegetables every day, the amount depending on the number of calories you require.

6) Your fruits and vegetables each day should include:
   1 serving *cruciferous vegetables* (cabbage, broccoli, etc.)
   1 serving *dark-green or dark-yellow vegetables* such as carrots or spinach
   1 serving of a *starchy vegetable* (corn, potatoes, peas, beans)
   1 serving *citrus fruit,* a six-ounce glass of fruit juice counts as one serving.

7) No matter how you distribute the rest of your fruits and vegetables throughout the day, you should eat a piece of fruit, or a serving of uncooked vegetables in a salad, *with every meal.*

8) You need at least *two slices of whole-grain* bread or the equivalent every day (for equivalents see page 186).

9) Keep alcohol consumption to a minimum, and skip it entirely now and then. Allow yourself one or at most two glasses of wine, cans of beer, or shots of whiskey each day, on all but the most special occasions.

10) Don't make heavily salt-cured, salt-pickled, or smoked foods a *major* part of your diet. But if you like them, you can enjoy them now and then.

A Day of Better Meals

Now let's examine how you can work these ideas into your existing mealtime habits. You probably eat three meals a day, with light snacks to keep you going. Most authorities believe it's best to spread your food intake fairly evenly throughout the day, but some people are inveterate breakfast-skippers or all-day nibblers (their bodies have gotten used to those idiosyncrasies.)

Breakfast

I used to be a strictly juice-and-coffee person in the morning; but I decided to try Dr. Denis Burkitt's policy of starting the day with a good dose of fiber, in the form of hot or cold whole-grain cereal. This bit of solid food at the outset has made me more energetic and productive in the early part of the day.

Breakfast is a good time for fresh fruit, either as juice or as

whole fruit. I usually have both. Fiber-rich cereal All-Bran o
granola in the warmer months; oatmeal or bulgur wheat
cooked in advance and heated in the morning in a double
boiler. I like to cut up an apple or a pear and toss it into the
cereal as it cooks. Or you can follow the Scandinavian cus
tom or *fruktost,* or "fruit-cheese," as the morning meal
Lean cheese; whole-grain bread, toast, or high-fiber flatbread
plus fresh fruit and coffee or tea makes a breakfast that'
satisfying but not heavy enough to slow you down. If you
simply must have eggs in the morning, use Egg Beaters, i
you think they're worth the money, or use one whole egg
plus one or two extra whites. Yes, you can have ham
sausage, or bacon—the much-reduced levels of nitrites and
nitrates that major meat packers now use lessen the cancer
risk significantly, and when you drink a big glass of orange
juice with your breakfast, the low levels of nitrite in the meat
are kept from oxidizing nitrosamines in your stomach.
Remember, though, that a hearty breakfast of this kind can
use up a hefty part of your day's calories, mostly in the form
of saturated fat.

Lunch

This is the meal most people eat away from home, when
we must depend either on cafeterias or restaurants or on food
brought with us. It's a meal where fat-calories can sneak in
unnoticed. Fortunately, more and more company cafeterias
and lower-priced restaurants are offering salad-bar service.
You can choose from a variety of fresh greens and vegetables,
a good low-fat, high-fiber basis for an everyday lunch. But
go easy on the dressing, which is usually oversalted and full
of so much oil or cheese that the good you do for yourself by
choosing salad in the first place can be undone. Better to
choose oil and vinegar, or take a couple of lemon wedges
from the tea counter and squeeze them on your salad at the
table. The typical fast-food lunch of a hamburger, combined
with cheese, lettuce, sauce, and other things on a white
hamburger roll, won't hurt you once in a while, but keep in
mind that a quarter-pounder gives you a total of 424 calories,
with 24 grams of fat, or 216 fat-calories!

For complete control over your midday meal, plus substantial savings, there's always the brown-bag lunch. The

xtra trouble it takes to pack your lunch in the morning before
etting out, or in the evening before a workday, is balanced
y not having to worry about extra fat creeping in undetected.
hese days, it seems that few people go to work or school
mpty-handed—we all seem to carry gym bags, attaché cases,
nd canvas totes. You might as well take along an interesting,
conomical, balanced lunch of foods that you really like.

You'll find a whole section on lunches to bring from home
n page 196. All of these suggestions fit right into the
alanced, varied, moderate, low-fat, high-fiber approach to
ating.

When a business associate invites you to lunch at a better-
han-everyday restaurant, you can choose between taking
ull luxurious advantages of your host's generosity (or the
ompany's expense account!), or sticking to your usual
ow-fat plan. It should depend, of course, on the way you
at the rest of the week and not on any foolish concerns
bout what people will think if you order an unconventional
meal.

You don't *have* to order a full entrée, which more often
than not gives you as much protein as you need for the whole
day, and more fat than you can use. These weight-watching
days, nobody gives it a second thought when you order a
large, plain green salad and the soup of the day, even at the
most posh of big-city restaurants. Beware of items on the
menu that *pretend* to be low in calories or fat and really
aren't. Chef's salad is an example—the five- or six-ounce
assortment of cheese strips and cold meats that usually tops
the bed of lettuce makes it a nice high-protein meal, with an
appreciable amount of fat, not the austere apology for a lunch
that many people want to believe.

When I'm taken out to lunch I look for à la carte vegetables:
my favorite broccoli or asparagus hollandaise, or artichokes
with vinaigrette sauce, or ratatouille, the wonderful garlicky
eggplant, tomato, and zucchini stew. Often I'll lunch on a
double portion of one of these vegetable dishes—with whole-
wheat bread and perhaps a dish of berries for dessert; it's a
lovely way to lunch, as elegant as can be, and a good
hollandaise sauce is a suitably special way to consume the
egg yolks and butter involved.

141

Dinner

The main meal of the day, for most families, and often the one time when everybody sits down together. It's a time for comfortable sharing, for relaxing together and reliving the day's events, when the pleasure of being together with the people you love the most should be reflected in the pleasure that the food provides. And if the day has been stressful and anxious, it's especially important for the pleasure of the dinner table to be as great as you can make it. An interesting meal can help take a person's mind off worries and problems. Familiar and beloved foods offer reassurance and security when the whole world seems to have gone wrong.

Meal planning requires sensitivity and imagination as much as a knowledge of nutrition and kitchen skills. When the children are studying hard for exams, or when the breadwinner is having a difficult time at work, it's hardly the best time to shock the family with an experimental dish. During stressful times, concentrate on conventional foods, unobtrusively supplemented: brownies laced with grated carrots, custard in which extra egg whites stand in for some of the yolks, the family's favorite stuffed peppers, with brown rice instead of white.

You'll probably be most successful in revising your eating habits if you reform them one step at a time. You could start quietly by putting a bowl of fresh fruit on the dinner table every night so that each member can help himself, even when traditional desserts are served. And do serve whole-grain bread with dinner. The more of this filling, fiber-rich food your family eats, the less fatty foods they'll want.

One good way to foster low-fat, high-fiber eating habits is to introduce new dishes combining meat and vegetables, such as stir-fried beef and vegetables, or using slightly more meat than is called for in the recipes on page 208. As time goes on and you repeat these dishes, gradually cut back on the meat and increase the proportion of vegetables.

You could also switch the emphasis of the evening meal from the standard meaty main dish to protein-rich before-dinner snacks of chicken wings, Hunan spicy beef, or tuna salad stuffed into cherry tomatoes, celery sticks, or slices of bell peppers, followed by a meal of vegetables, soups, grain dishes, and fruit. After an introductory course of meat, fish, or poultry, interestingly prepared, you might serve assorted steamed vegetables (celery, broccoli, zucchini, red-pepper strips, carrots, potatoes, onions, served with a sauce of lemon juice, Worcestershire sauce, and beef broth). Or a similar assortment of steamed vegetables that have been marinated in a garlic-flavored white wine, olive oil, and mustard dressing. Or a baked vegetable casserole.

Or, after a fish or liver pâté, serve a hearty soup (leek and potato, mushroom barley, or ad hoc vegetable) plus a generous salad of mixed greens, cold leftover vegetables, and low-fat dressing. Serving meat separately will encourage you and your family to think about meat as something special, to be savored, not as a bulky food to be taken for granted and wolfed down.

Small alterations in the way you eat will help you cut down somewhat on the fat in your diet, bring more friendly fiber to your table, increase your intake of micronutrients and protective compounds, and reduce your exposure to some of the more worrisome substances.

What's more, they will start you *thinking* in a high-fiber, low-fat, anticancer mode. Taking a minute to disrobe a chicken of its fatty skin reinforces your knowledge that fat is not your friend. Reaching for the whole-wheat crackers on the supermarket shelf reminds you that fiber, in any form, is a vital part of your diet.

As I adopted them, I noticed my attitudes changing. Trimming the fat from my meat has become an automatic dinnertable ritual, like putting my napkin in my lap. And I notice when other people fail to push the fat to the side of their plates. What's the matter with them? Don't they *know* how important it is?

Choosing fruit instead of ice cream used to be an agonizing, self-denying act, until a few special occasions, when I treated myself to a rich dessert and realized that grapefruit is not forever, it's for every day. If I follow the fruit-for-dessert strategy as a rule, it's okay for me to eat something sinful now and then.

Once you start thinking this way, it's an easy step to the balanced, varied, moderate diet implicit in the NAS committee's guidelines. And you may decide to move on to the more systematic approach of the Everyday Food Plans, beginning on page 177.

All of us can start, in our kitchens and supermarkets, at our dinner tables and in the line at the cafeteria, to bring our diet into line with the facts that are known right now.

- We can start eating the number of calories we need. No more.
- We can cut out a quarter of the calories we get from fat by choosing lean cuts of meat and trimming the fat away.
- We can increase the amount of fiber, vitamin C, beta-carotene, inhibitors of carcinogenesis, and trace minerals by eating goodly amounts of fruits, whole grains, and vegetables—especially the cruciferae.
- We can make up for the fat calories we've eliminated by eating more of the carbohydrate foods we've been avoiding all these years, and by getting to know some of the fat-free protein-rich foods we've been unaware of.
- We can bring our liquor consumption down to sensible levels, and if we're still smoking, we can abstain from alcohol altogether.
- We can keep our consumption of extra-salty ethnic foods *down*.
- We can avoid heavily smoked foods most of the time.
- We can go lightly on nitrate- and nitrite-cured processed meats.
- We can minimize the amount of saccharin and diet soda we consume, or better still, eliminate the stuff entirely.
- We can start reading the labels on packaged and processed foods before we buy them, using fewer of those containing a lot of additives.
- We can reserve for special occasions the foods we know are rich in mutagens.

The way you choose to go about it is up to you.

Your Food Diary

To help yourself get started on your new way of eating, it's a good idea to get a little notebook for your pocket or purse and write down what you eat—down to the last handful of peanuts—and the quantity, as nearly as you can estimate it.

Consult your Nutrition Counter frequently and jot down the number of calories you consume each day. Make a special note of how much of each of the three types of fats you eat every day.

For the first few weeks, you should keep a fairly detailed record. A day's food diary might read:

Breakfast:
> ½ grapefruit, 2 slices whole-grain toast, 1 tsp. butter, coffee, ½ cup low-fat milk.

Coffee Break:
> Bran muffin, coffee, low-fat milk.

Lunch:
> Grilled-cheese sandwich (whole-wheat bread, 1 oz. Swiss cheese), 1 cup mixed greens with vinegar and 1 tsp. olive oil, ½ cup fresh mixed fruit, diet soda.

Snack:
> Carrot sticks, ½ cup apple juice.

Dinner:
> 4 oz. lean hamburger, broiled; ½ cup green peas; 1 cup coleslaw (low-fat dressing); 1 baked apple (with 2 tsps. honey); 1 glass white wine.

Snack:
> Small slice carrot cake.

Total Calories for Day: 2,400

Later, when you feel your new attitudes toward food and your reshaped habits are well-established, you may need only a rough daily total of calories and notes of significant deviations—good or bad—from your balanced, varied, moderate way of life.

A week's jottings in your food diary at a later stage could run something like this:

Sunday:

1,100 calories approx. Vegetarian day. 2 tsp. olive oil, 1 teaspoon margarine. No alcohol. Cold pasta, bean soup for dinner.

Monday:

1,800 calories approx. Whole egg for breakfast. No cruciferae. 2 glasses light beer. Tried oatmeal bread, not bad for first attempt.

Tuesday:

2,100 calories approx. Coleslaw, lunch. Brussels sprouts, dinner. Tried shredded carrots in meat loaf for dinner—need more onion.

Wednesday:

1,500 calories approx. Glass red wine with dinner.

Thursday:

1,500 calories. Skipped breakfast. Big lunch at Smokey's barbecue. Ribs! Cabbage salad for dinner, lots of carrot sticks.

Friday:

1,200 calories (vegetarian). Tried for lowest possible fat.

> *Breakfast:* Juice, bulgur wheat with stewed prunes, black coffee.
>
> *Lunch:* Steamed vegetables with brown rice, chicken broth with noodles and broccoli, peaches.
>
> *Dinner:* Low-fat ratatouille (great!), ricotta cheese with leftover vegetables, zucchini bread, fresh pineapple. "Cappucino" with low-fat milk tastes just like the real thing.

Saturday:

2,000 calories. Omelette (1 whole egg plus Egg Beaters). 4 oz. prime filet mignon (!). Extra coleslaw.

Sunday:

1,100 calories. Vegetarian day—mostly fruit. Dash of Liquid Smoke in baked beans for dinner, good idea.

And so forth.

You'll find it helpful to note the family's reactions to new recipes—I experimented with stars and exclamation points and finally hit upon using a circle, with two dots for eyes, and a mouth line that curved upward in a smile, beside foods that went over well, and a turned-down mouth for foods nobody liked much. Such a food diary adds to the spirit of adventure in eating, and as the weeks pass and the smilers and ''yuck''-faces accumulate, you and your family will begin to feel a greater sense of involvement with your healthier way of eating. The record of what you've been eating will sharpen your awareness—it was by keeping a food diary that included my snacks as well as regular meals that I discovered how conveniently I'd been ignoring the quantity of cheese I had been eating.

17
The Food Groups

When we look at the foods we eat, it's more practical, more correct scientifically, and much easier to keep things straight, if we divide foods into categories. It's certainly less trouble than trying to impose an artificial calorie-counting system on our eating habits.

The four main food groups are made up of nutritionally important foods:

I.   Milk, milk products, and cheese
II. Grains, breads, and cereals
III. Meat, fish, poultry, and eggs
IV. Vegetables and fruits

The luxury foods—fats, sugars, and alcohol—are more significant for the enjoyment they add when used in sensible amounts, and for the problems they cause when we overindulge, than for nutritional value, since for practical purposes these are low-nutrient, high-calorie foods. They're considered separately.

Let's look at each food group carefully, it terms of the ordinary, wholesome foods we eat, giving special attention to those that can increase or decrease your risks of cancer.

Group I. Milk, Milk Products, and Cheese

Nutritionists are worried about the relatively low amounts of milk, yogurt, and cheese that seem to be standard with many American adults, since this food group is the main source of calcium and riboflavin in the diet. One reason many of us consume too little food from the dairy department may be that we consider it all right for babies, but not for ourselves—not realizing that without the calcium provided by milk and milk products, our bones will grow brittle, a condition known as *osteoporosis*.

We may also stay away from milk and related foods because we've heard that they contain fat, particularly saturated fat.

The changing dietary habits of Americans have not been lost on the dairy industry, who have responded with a wide range of products from which all or part of the fat has been removed. About the only product they haven't developed yet is fat-free butter, and now there's a butter-margarine blend.

Reduced-fat dairy products vary in their similarity to the "real" thing; as substitutes, some of them are dismal, but as low-fat foods they are fine.

Milk. Eight ounces of whole milk contains 8.1 grams of fat—5.1 grams of saturated fat, 0.3 grams of polyunsaturated fat, and 33 milligrams of cholesterol. Skim milk, with nonfat milk solids added to give it body, contains only .6 grams of fat, .4 grams of which is saturated, and only 5 milligrams of cholesterol. For cooking purposes, and as a drink, the skim milk performs just as well as the whole milk.

With milk that is 1 percent or 2 percent fat, the percentages refer to the proportion of fat in the milk, not that these types of milk contain only a small percentage of the fat contained in whole milk. "One percent fat milk," for example, contains a total of 2.4 grams of fat per eight-ounce serving.

Low-Fat Cheeses. Part-skim mozzarella, low-fat processed cheeses, imitation cream cheese, and the dairy industry's other answers to the need for low-fat high-protein foods are mainstays in my refrigerator. A nice imported low-fat cheese is the mild and creamy-tasting Swiss Lace—served, of course, with my cheese scraper. Neufchatel is a spreadable low-fat delight. I keep a chunk of good Parmesan for grating, but I use it sparingly, just for flavor. Be warned—low-fat cheeses don't melt as satisfactorily as the originals.

Sour Cream. With only about 2.5 grams of fat per tablespoonful, it's a relatively harmless touch of luxury. Try two tablespoonfuls on piping hot green beans sprinkled with a little dried basil.

Yogurt. Plain yogurt has 3.5 grams of fat per eight-ounce container. Mix it half-and-half with sour cream in recipes calling for the cream in large quantities. Yogurt is one of the best meat tenderizers there is—use it to marinate the low-fat cuts of beef which are likely to be tough. It's also a good foundation for sauces and salad dressings, combining the tartness of vinegar or lemon juice with the body otherwise provided by oils. If you add seasonings to yogurt—fresh or dried herbs; minced garlic and grated lemon peel; curry powder or other spices—you've got a quick and easy low-fat sauce.

If you object to the sour taste, add a smidge of sugar or honey, *after* you've mixed the yogurt-based sauce or dressing with the ingredients you'll be serving it with. The acidity is toned down naturally by the flavor of other ingredients.

Fruit-flavored yogurt has even less fat per eight-ounce container—2.4 grams—but you pay for it with calories from sugar.

Ice Cream. Save it for super-special occasions; it contains 7.2 grams of fat in a half-cup serving.

Ice Milk. It's just as delicious as ice cream, with only 2.8 grams of fat per serving. If your family resists, try serving ice milk with new and exciting toppings (cranberry-orange relish spooned over vanilla ice milk is one of the world's great desserts, and I'll bet you haven't tried it).

Cream. A once-in-a-great-while treat—on the first fresh raspberries of the year, for example. Use 2 percent fat milk in your coffee, a small change in flavor you'll get used to quickly. Avoid powdered cream substitutes—they're *loaded* with saturated fats from coconut or palm oil, and offer no advantage.

Group II. Grains, Breads, and Cereal

Whole grains are a splendid source of the pentosan fraction of fiber—the kind that may have the most potent anticancer powers. Most Americans and Western Europeans don't eat enough fiber of any kind, as our high colon-cancer incidence attests.

Happily, whole grains are delicious, versatile, good sources of carbohydrates and of protein, too, when combined correctly with other foods, and the interesting textures and filling properties of whole grains make meatless meals satisfying and enjoyable. One of the kinds of whole grain that is easiest to introduce into the average family diet is *bulgur wheat*—coarsely ground whole wheat that works well in stuffings, casseroles, and hearty salads, but is glamorous enough to stand alone as a side dish with roast beef, fish, turkey, or other family favorites.

Brown rice is a supermarket item available everywhere, and like bulgur, a good starchy side dish. Where possible, try to use brown rice instead of the white kind. *Oatmeal*—the old-fashioned kind that takes a while to cook—contains more protein than any grain in everyday use. It is, of course, a wintertime favorite for breakfast, and a good alternative to a bacon and eggs breakfast. I often use oatmeal as a substitute for bread crumbs, in meat loaf, meatballs, and as a topping for casseroles.

Less well-known grains deserve a place in your diet, too. *Barley* is delicious and as easy to prepare as rice; a transitional alternative to white rice if your family is too conservative for a sudden switch to brown rice. *Wild rice* is expensive, but I think it's the most delicious of all the whole grains, and I always have some on hand. It adds a nice touch to the savory whole-grain side dish I call hot granola, or other whole-grain combinations, and it can stand alone as the centerpiece of an otherwise frugal meatless meal.

Bread and other baked goods are made from ground grain flour. White "enriched" flour, as you surely know, is made from the starchy, nutrient-poor part of the wheat, the good fiber gone forever, with a pathetic fraction of the lost vitamins and minerals restored artifically later in the process. Sadly, most of our most familiar baked foods are based on white flour; you just can't make white bread or an angel food cake from whole-wheat flour.

For old favorites, where nothing else will do, I use white flour, the "unbleached" kind, as snowy as ordinary flour but with a little more of the vitamins. I use it in foods where I want to have the traditional color and texture; for light and elegant cakes I take out one tablespoonful of the unbleached flour (which is a little too heavy for a feather-light result) from each cupful and replace it with a tablespoonful of cornstarch before sifting.

Most of the time, however, I use a combination of unbleached flour plus whole wheat. When making gingerbread or any kind of dark-colored cake or cookie, I mix unbleached and whole-wheat flour in equal proportions without sifting. And for bread, as you can see from the recipes, I use a combination of flours.

Bran, strictly speaking, is not a whole grain—it's the fibrous outer coating of the wheat berry. I use bran often in baking, and I sneak it into all kinds of foods to add the benefits of fiber. Bran is one of the cheapest foods you can buy, it contains no calories, has little flavor of its own, and is wonderfully high in pentose.

I add a tablespoonful to every pound of ground beef I use, and to every batch of brownies. If I have to use a cake mix instead of baking from scratch, a tablespoonful goes into the batter. With a rich traditional meal, with butter and eggs and all the special-occasion ingredients, I'm careful to add bran wherever I can—a tablespoonful or two in the dressing for the turkey, another tablespoonful in the mincemeat for the pie, a dusting of bran added to the bread-crumb-and-butter topping for the creamed onions. Nobody notices, but I have the quiet satisfaction of knowing that along with all the fat, my loved ones are eating pentosan fiber, too.

Table 1. The Fiber in Grains, Breads, and Cereals

Type of Grain	Amount	Grams of Fiber
Plain miller's bran	½ cup	6.6
Oatmeal (cooked)	1 cup	1.9
60% whole-wheat bread	1 slice	1.4
100% whole-grain bread	1 slice	2.4
Boiled rice (white)	½ cup	0.8
White "enriched" bread	1 slice	0.7
All Bran	½ cup	12.0
Shredded Wheat	2 biscuits	6.2
Bran Flakes	1 cup	4.8
Rice Krispies	1 cup	1.4

Group III. Meat, Fish, Poultry, and Eggs

Meat. When shopping for meat for everyday meals, choose not only the leanest cuts but the individual packages that have the least fat. Look for beef that's plain, bright red—those white flecks of fat, known as marbling, that you see in the most expensive cuts are symbols of the high-fat diet that adds to our colon-cancer risk. Look for the cheaper grades which, by law, have less marbling.

Antifat guru Nathan Pritikin recommends commercial grade beef, the cheapest of all. It's not very tender, but if cooked slowly it loses much of its toughness, and has a good beefy flavor. But commercial-grade beef is hard to find. "Good," the next grade up on the scale, is often sold in supermarkets, sometimes labeled as "lean."

The meat producers, who are as profit-minded as anyone, have been listening to their market researchers and know that everybody these days wants to cut down on fat. So most of the meat now sold comes from animals bred to be leaner than in the past. This is particularly true of pork. If you trim the visible fat away from supermarket pork chops or fresh ham, the meat you end up with is no fattier than good lean beef.

Except for country-cured ham, bacon, and sausage, the amounts of nitrites and nitrates now used in processed meats are very low indeed—much lower than they were when worries about nitrosamines surfaced in the mid-1970's. Ham and cold cuts from major meat packers nowadays do not pose a nitrite threat to anybody, though it makes sense to vary your diet and not eat processed or cured meats every day. But the same products from small companies, backwoods smokehouses, and local concerns may be made from the old-fashioned recipes, which call for high levels of sodium nitrate (saltpeter). Be cautious about these foods.

When it's time to celebrate, or when it just seems the moment for a conventionally luxurious meal, I like to go first class. I shop for the prime rib roast, the tenderest lamb. My feeling is that since I don't do this every day, I want meat that is, by classic standards, the best. I do keep the portions moderate—not stingy, but not overwhelming. That's okay, because we're going for quality tonight.

A four- or five-ounce serving of the best beef fillet, prepared with exquisite care and served as part of a lovingly planned meal is, I believe, more luxurious than a full-pound steak of mediocre quality, served in a slapdash manner. More, I feel, isn't necessarily better.

On other occasions when company comes, I may serve a leaner, less conventionally lavish feast to them. I plan and prepare it with the same care I put into a rich meal, and observe the principles of balance, variety, and moderation. The finger foods on the cocktail table are raw vegetables, neatly trimmed and arranged attractively with a yogurt-and-spice dip, or chick-peas mashed with garlic, lemon juice, and lots of pepper. The meal itself is low in fat, with broccoli, brussels sprouts, or cabbage in some form, a loaf of home-made bread, low-fat cheese and a fruit tray for dessert. There's meat, fish, or poultry in decent amounts, but the rest of the meal is so interesting that my guests eat enough of everything else, and they don't have to fill up on the meat. I serve wine for those who like it, but I let people help them-selves and don't force them to take more than they want.

(And I never call attention to the fact that this is a meal consciously planned to conform to my lower-cancer-risk strategy. After all, this is a party.)

Fish. A first-class source of protein, with little waste and not much fat. Broil or poach for the greatest savings in fat-calories. Sometimes, I think we consider fish a calorie-free food, but it's not. A four-ounce portion is plenty.

And canned fish, like tuna or sardines packed in oil, can undo your efforts to cut down on fat. For tuna salad, I use only tuna packed in water, and when using sardines or anchovies, I'm careful to drain them well and rinse them under the cold water tap.

Once in a while I buy the Italian tuna packed in olive oil, and use it in a salade Niçoise: romaine lettuce, thawed frozen green beans, tomato wedges, tiny boiled potatoes in their skins, a light dressing of lemon juice and Dijon mustard, with that magnificent tuna—its olive oil mostly drained away. I top it with red onion rings and lots of freshly ground black pepper and serve it with whole-grain bread and a little low-fat cheese.

That's a pretty elegant meal.

Freshly caught fish from lakes and streams is one of the

great delights of the table, but these days many people worry about the chemicals that freshwater fish may pick up from polluted waters. The NAS committee did not see a danger, so far as cancer is concerned. If you like your catfish and your crawdads, go ahead and enjoy them, but keep in mind the protective principles—don't eat them every day, consume cancer-inhibiting foods along with them, and make sure you're eating a balanced, varied, and moderate diet as a way of life.

Poultry. Where would we be without chicken? It's tasty, inexpensive, and versatile. Almost everybody loves it. It's one of the best sources of protein, and when the skin and yellow clumps of fat are removed, chicken is not only one of the leanest meats available, the little fat that does remain is largely unsaturated.

But don't focus exclusively on chicken. Other forms of poultry are available in your supermarket, and in keeping with the principle of varying your food choices, pay due attention to turkey (whole, in parts, chopped, or as processed meats), and game hens.

Cooking a whole turkey is a bit of a chore, but the cooked bird usually lasts for several meals. In theory, it's desirable to skin the turkey before cooking, but in my experience this is not only a good deal of trouble, it leads to a dried-out bird that becomes even more dehydrated after a day in the refrigerator. I peel the cooked skin away from each portion after cooking, and leave the skin on the leftover carcass to keep the moisture in.

Game hens are lovely, but most are really too big for one person and not quite enough for two. I solve this by removing the legs before cooking and serving one legless bird per person, saving the legs for another meal. Like chicken, game hens should be skinned before cooking.

Large or small, whole birds are nicest when they're stuffed with some savory mixture. I always rub the inside cavity with ground ginger, whatever the rest of the stuffing consists of—ginger seems to do something special for the flavor.

Instead of stuffings based on white bread or bread crumbs, I like to substitute brown rice or bulgur wheat. The taste is much the same when onions and herbs are added, but the texture is more interesting and the healthy fiber and micronutrients make the stuffing more worth eating.

155

One of my favorite poultry stuffings consists of equal parts of cooked brown rice and chopped frozen spinach (thawed), with minced onion, garlic, and fresh dill to taste, and chunks of feta cheese. This combination also works beautifully as stuffing for a whole fish, baked or broiled. All-vegetable stuffings (chopped broccoli, mixed with grated carrots, chopped onions, and celery, for example) make an extra-low-fat meal seem special.

Most recipes calling for chicken parts begin by browning the chicken in oil or butter. If you're not careful, this can more than make up for the intrinsically low fat content in the poultry. When you brown, always use a mixture of saturated, monounsaturated, and polyunsaturated fats (I like butter, corn oil, and peanut oil in equal parts), and after browning, pour all the liquid out of the pan. If the next step in the recipe requires the fat left over from browning the chicken, use the thin film clinging to the pan—it's usually enough to cook the onions or heat the curry powder to do whatever else needs to be done, provided you stir carefully and keep the heat low. If you are worried that there is too little fat in the pan to prevent burning, pour in a few tablespoons of white wine—or even beer!—stir, heat, and proceed as if you were following the recipe. The results will be indistinguishable to most people, though those with superfine palates may notice that the vegetable ingredients have a slightly softer texture than when cooked in the conventional way.

Eggs. A fine source of protein, and the yolks have a way of emulsifying fats in other foods so they integrate with other ingredients to make a smooth and flavorful blend. But the yolks contain 64 calories and a lot of them come from saturated fat and cholesterol. Though the NAS committee has no specific recommendation on eggs, other authorities warn us not to eat too many yolks. The American Health Foundation says that two or three egg yolks per week is enough for an adult; the USDA allows three or four.

Use them well, in hollandaise and other sauces, or as the boiled or fried eggs you crave for breakfast. There are times when nothing but a whole egg will do. But there are many other occasions when we use whole eggs just because we're used to doing so, not because the yolk is really necessary, and at those times you can make creative substitutions.

156

One is Egg Beaters, the frozen egg substitute which is really just egg whites, colored with beta-carotene and flavored with a little salt. They're very convenient but rather expensive. Dr. John H. Weisburger, director of the American Health Foundation, tells me that he makes omelettes for his family every Saturday morning, using one whole egg plus a container of Egg Beaters. The Belgian-born Dr. Weisburger has high standards for food, and assures me that these low-fat omelettes are indistinguishable from the traditional kind. Well, we disagree, but try them yourself.

For a two-egg omelette or serving of scrambled eggs, I prefer the natural taste and the greater economy of using one whole egg plus one or two extra whites. It's not as yellow as a regular omelette, but the taste is the same. (Try adding a little flaked leftover fish, or coarsely grated orange peel to scrambled eggs for a refreshing change.)

In cakes, cookies, meat loaf, and hundreds of other dishes calling for eggs, you can substitute three egg whites for every two whole eggs. Where one whole egg is called for, use one egg white plus a tablespoonful of polyunsaturated vegetable oil.

Group IV. Fruits and Vegetables

Vegetables

Your supermarket is a treasury of fresh fruits and vegetables throughout the year. Don't let yourself get into a rut, buying the same assortment every time you do your marketing —explore, experiment, and make the most of the bounty that's offered!

Wash these items thoroughly. The NAS committee says that any amounts of pesticides or contaminants clinging to our food is probably so small that it cannot affect our cancer risk, but just as a matter of simple sanitation, washing is important. (I know a woman who's so displeased by the oil that her produce store rubs on the skin of cucumbers to make them shiny that she washes her cucumbers with soap and water—an unnecessary extreme.)

Eat the skins and seeds whenever possible—they contain wonderful fiber and perhaps other important compounds. Of course, some parts of some fruits and vegetables are just too much to cope with—the skin of a pineapple, the stem of an eggplant. But you'd be surprised how much you can salvage from fresh foods—those tough parts at the core of a cabbage, chopped fine, can go into soup; simmered along with the potatoes and carrots for an hour or so, they add body and depth of flavor. Broccoli stems require peeling; stripped of the tough outer sheath and cut in slices a quarter inch thick, the stems are tender enough to serve along with the florets, or mixed with carrot strips of the same size and thickness.

Score the skins of an unpeeled cucumber lengthwise with the tines of a fork before you slice it for a salad; this renders the skin less chewy and gives it a decorative appearance.

Fruits

Like vegetables, fruits provide a wide range of fiber, and are naturally low in sodium. They are among the best sources of vitamin C. They make convenient, tasty snacks and desserts. But fruits contain high levels of sugars, which mean calories. You can't eat unlimited amounts of sweet, juicy fruit and stay within your calorie allowance. Fruit is *food*.

Citrus fruits. Oranges, grapefruit, lemons, limes, tangelos, tangerines, kumquats, and those odd-looking but delicious "uggli" fruits are rich sources of vitamin C. For this reason, the NAS committee guidelines call special attention to this family of fruits.

Deep-yellow fruits. This type includes peaches, apricots, nectarines, cantaloupe, mangoes, and papaya. They are splendid sources of beta-carotene.

Melons. They, too, are excellent sources of vitamin C. Cantaloupes, particularly, are important to anyone who wants to get the most protection against cancer from good everyday foods, for they provide vitamin A, as well. Have you tried cantaloupe with fresh ginger, one of those classic combinations of flavors? Grate a little ginger over plain cantaloupe, or serve cantaloupe with a mound of vanilla ice milk or low-fat cottage cheese, a gilding of shredded ginger on top.

Berries. A source of vitamin C in lavish amounts. They come in so many varieties, as the seasons progress, that during the spring and summer you can concentrate on one kind after another: the strawberries of spring, the raspberries of June and July, blackberries in August. Nowadays, most supermarkets offer cultivated blueberries and strawberries the year round. They're pretty but rather flavorless out of season, I think, and are most useful in adding a touch of color and luxury to winter desserts of mixed fruit. (Orange and grapefruit sections, with unpeeled apples, cut in chunks, sprinkled with a little rum, kirsch, or frozen orange juice contentrate, acquire a dressier look when you add a handful of blueberries or sliced strawberries.)

In season, fresh, locally grown berries are worth celebrating. Arrange flawless strawberries, washed but with the stems left on, on your prettiest plates, a ring of berries surrounding a tiny mound of sifted confectioners' sugar (a teaspoonful or two is all you need).

Sliced and sweetened, if necessary, with a little sugar, honey, or liqueur, and spooned over a simple cake (angel food, sponge, or store-bought pound cake), berries make an elegant dessert with a sense of importance—just right for a company dinner or family occasion.

Your supermarket or corner produce store has a bountiful array of other fruits, of course. Sample all of them and make them a part of your balanced, varied, moderate diet, but try to include some citrus fruit, melon, or berries in your diet every day to make sure you get the vitamin C you need.

Fruit juice. A convenient way to get your citrus fruit, particularly, but remember that juices contain virtually no fiber, and the squeezing and straining may eliminate other important substances as well. Most canned and many frozen fruit juices contain added sugar—read the labels! Those sold as "fruit drinks" or "punch" are the most sugary—unless you're a real addict and compensate for the sugar by cutting down elsewhere in your diet, avoid these products.

Canned and frozen fruits. Most are packed in sugar syrup, which may occupy a surprisingly large proportion of the container. When you drain the liquid away, there's always less fruit than you expect, and it's soggy with sugar. And it's expensive!

If for some reason you *want* canned or frozen fruit, buy the kind without added sugar—canned in water or in its own juice, frozen without syrup. I find it's much more convenient to serve *fresh* fruit—the only preparation it requires is a good wash, and there's no container to throw away.

Thin-skinned fruits like apples and pears, whose peel has no objectionable flavor, don't need to be peeled, whether they're eaten whole as a snack or in a cup of fruit mélange.

Table 2. The Fiber in Fruits

Fruit	Amount	Grams of Fiber
Cherries	1 cup	2.0
Peach (with skin)	1 medium	2.1
Orange	1 medium	2.3
Raisins	¼ cup	2.7
Apple (with skin)	1 medium	4.0

Vegetables

All vegetables provide fiber of various types, especially if you eat them with their skins and seeds. Although many of the cruciferae (cabbage family) belong in the dark-green vegetable category, they are listed here as a separate group to give them the extra emphasis they deserve because of their carcinogenesis-inhibiting properties.

Everybody needs *at least three* servings of vegetables each day. Though you might want to make all your servings consist of nothing but your favorite vegetable, it's much better to vary your choices. Broccoli is good for you, but so are all the others. Try to eat at least one dark-green, one deep-yellow, and one cruciferous vegetable each day. And if you are a smoker, lean heavily on the ones that provide the most beta-carotene.

A. Dark-green and deep-yellow vegetables are fine sources of vitamin A. Those that are dark green are all high in fiber, low in calories, and good sources of vitamin C, folacin, iron, and magnesium.

Dark Green	Deep-Yellow
Spinach	Carrots
Broccoli	Winter squash
Green peppers	Acorn squash
Chicory	Pumpkin
Endive	Sweet Potatoes
Escarole	Yams
Romaine lettuce	
Watercress	
Greens:	

Greens:
Kale	Beet
Turnip	Dandelion
Mustard	Swiss chard

Dark-green vegetables include many of the cruciferae, so when you serve broccoli, kale, turnip greens, and the others, you get two different kinds of benefits at the same time.

Chopped, frozen spinach is a great convenience for any cook. A good simple vegetable when served along with a dab of margarine or sour cream, it's an admirable "stretcher" for ground meat, a colorful bit of contrast in a side dish of whole grains, an imaginative ingredient to add to a sauce that seems to lack character, and a welcome addition to a vegetable soup that seems a little too thin.

Deep-yellow Vegetables

Carrots are a vegetable you can serve at any meal (carrot muffins or pancakes for breakfast!) or as a low-calorie snack any time of day; they're your best source of beta-carotene.

Some people don't like the taste of raw carrots, and if that's a problem with your family, serve carrots in other ways. You might grate up a bunch next time you're using your food processor (or grate them by hand; it doesn't take long) and keep them in a covered plastic container in the refrigerator. When the inspiration strikes you, you can toss a handful into whatever you're cooking. Add them to salads, cookies, casseroles, and sauces. Sprinkle them as a garnish. Stir them into meat dishes as a stretcher. Grated carrots are nice added to gingerbread or chocolate cake. A cup of grated carrots provides the equivalent of more than three times the minimum daily requirement for vitamin A.

Don't forget that squash and pumpkin, too, are excellent sources of beta-carotene. A cup of pumpkin pulp from a can equals *twelve times* the minimum daily requirement for vitamin A. Left whole, these amusing vegetables lend themselves to being stuffed with other things. Cut acorn squash in half horizontally and remove the seeds, then cut a thin slice off each end so that it can stand up without wobbling. Boil for 25 minutes, or until soft but not squishy, and you have attractive shells to fill with mixed vegetables (broccoli, diced potatoes, and red pepper), whole grains (cooked wheat berries and diced apples, sprinkled with honey and cinnamon), or a meat filling (ground lean pork, chopped cabbage and onions, bound with mashed carrots and moistened with cider).

A medium-sized pumpkin, hollowed out and boiled whole for 45 minutes, makes a spectacular container for a stew. I sprinkle the inside with beef bouillon powder after it's cooked, put the pumpkin in a Pyrex pie plate, and fill it with beef stew or a lamb curry, then replace the top portion of the pumpkin as a lid. You ladle out each person's portion of stew, then cut pieces of the pumpkin "tureen" for each.

B. Starchy vegetables contribute fiber, protein, iron, zinc, magnesium, phosphorus, thiamine, vitamin B_6, and folacin, as well as the starch that makes them filling and a good fat-free calorie source.

Potatoes:	Parsnips
White	Rutabagas
Sweet	Yams
Dried Peas and Beans:	Plantains
Lentils	Lima beans
Chick-peas	Green peas
Split peas	Corn
Navy beans	
Black beans	
Black-eyed peas	

Potatoes. People used to think that potatoes were fattening, but now we realize that it's what we do to them that makes us

162

fat, not the 150 calories we get in a plain baked Idaho. One french fry has 14 calories and half a gram of fat, frozen baked potatoes with cheese and other adornments have over 300 calories! Potatoes are tasty, and among the best sources of trace minerals, particularly chromium, so we should use a little imagination about serving them. It doesn't make sense to serve fat-enriched potatoes with an already rich meal unless it's a special occasion.

One of my favorite treats is a kingly baked potato, topped with a tablespoon of sour cream, a bit of grated onion—and a spoonful of *caviar*! In the spring, when tiny new potatoes about as big as strawberries are available in some stores I serve them this way, as hot accompaniments to a drink before a super-special dinner. (Yes, caviar is heavily salt-cured, but I don't think anyone has ever eaten enough to show whether it could affect cancer risk!)

Besides the obvious ways of serving potatoes—as ingredients in soups and stews, mashed (with low-fat milk or yogurt) as a side dish, or boiled in their skins, consider serving them in unfamiliar ways. Line individual baking dishes with mashed potatoes, sprinkle with paprika and brown in the oven, and fill them with flaked fish in a dill-flecked sauce. Or boil big potatoes split in half, scoop out the middle, and fill with beef bourguignon.

Sweet potatoes and yams. They provide all the virtues of the white varieties, and a hefty bonus of beta-carotene, as well. They don't have to be smothered with marshmallows or brown sugar to be delectable. My mother used to make a very simple casserole of cooked yams, cut in chunks, quartered apples, and strips of lean smoked ham, baked, covered, in a 350-degree oven for 40 minutes, which never failed to please. She sprinkled a little powdered cloves on top. You could substitute strips of lean fresh pork and add a half teaspoonful of Liquid Smoke, or you could use nitrite-free sausage, browned and drained.

Though it's not at all authentic, I like to serve mashed sweet potatoes, thinned with yogurt and spiced with grated fresh ginger and nutmeg, with an Indian meal—it's a nice foil for this and other spicy dishes.

Legumes. These are members of the bean family—peas, lentils, and beans of all kinds and colors: pink, black, white, lima, navy, pinto, and Great Northern. Their subdued flavors make them good companions for authoritative seasonings and strongly flavored foods. When combined with grains, which have certain amino acids that legumes lack, beans and their relatives make good, complete protein meals without meat. A feast of rice and beans, a dish of pasta and beans, or a dinner of lentil soup with whole-grain bread provides you with all the protein you need, at a cost of very few fat calories. These grain plus legume combinations are the foundations of solid peasant fare in many countries, where meat of any kind is a rare treat. (See the Trade-Offs, page 186, for exact proportions.)

If you haven't cooked much with beans in the past, start with a couple of cans of plain red kidney beans and garbanzos (chick-peas) and try one of the bean recipes in Chapter 19. Though a bit mushy in texture, canned beans taste fine and are already cooked. Dried legumes, even the quick-cooking kind, require long boiling.

Bean curd. An Oriental achievement—soybean solids compressed in a smooth, bland cake with the consistency of soft cheese. Available at Oriental and health food stores and at some supermarkets, bean curd is a very versatile means of stretching costlier forms of protein (I've been known to add it to seafood salad when more people showed up for a luncheon party than I'd planned for). Whirled in a blender with lemon juice, seasonings, and a touch of oil, it makes a smooth and creamy salad dressing. Its amino acids complement those of rice to make Oriental vegetarian dishes good sources of protein.

C. Cruciferae contain indoles and many other compounds, and among them are substances that have a cancer-inhibiting effect. These vegetables also contain fiber, and most contain vitamins A and C, a variety of minerals, and few calories. They include:

Cabbage:	Mustard greens
White	Swiss chard
Red	Kale
Savoy	Cauliflower:
Napa	White
Bok choy	Purple
Kohlrabi	Broccoli
Turnip greens	Brussels sprouts

Some people object to the strong cabbagey flavor of these vetetables, but there are ways around it. Avoid overcooking, and where possible, cook in a steamer or a rack over boiling water and remove the vegetable from the heat while it's still crisp.

For a total absence of cabbagey taste, serve these vegetables raw, in salads or as crudités. Chopped white cabbage, carrots, and crushed pineapple make a salad even little kids love. Mix chopped Savoy cabbage leaves into soups or sauces during the last five minutes of cooking—I sometimes do this with spaghetti sauce, and it's wonderful!

D. Other vegetables contribute different nutrients, and add variety to your menus. Eat a wide range of vegetables in season to make sure you don't miss out on vitamins, minerals, or trace nutrients. Try some of the following:

Tomatoes	Artichokes
Eggplant	Asparagus
Peppers	Okra
Beets	Mushrooms
Fresh Beans	Radishes
Green	Cucumbers
Yellow	Turnips
Purple	Squash
Onions	Summer
White	Butternut
Yellow	Spaghetti
Red	Zucchini
Green (scallions)	
Lettuce	
Iceberg	
Leaf	
Bibb	
Celery	

You don't really need to peel carrots, squash, potatoes, and the like. Just wash well, scrubbing if necessary. Tomatoes can also go unpeeled when they're served raw, but when cooked, their skins become tough and curl into unpleasant little shreds, so I like to remove the skins by dipping the tomatoes into boiling water before cooking. Tomato seeds can be removed easily when the vegetable is raw—I use my thumb to ease them out—but this is necessary only for very exacting classic recipes. Most people don't object to the seeds of tomatoes, and may enjoy the texture and touch of flavor.

Table 3. The Fiber in Vegetables

Vegetable	Amount	Grams of Fiber
Lettuce (raw)	1 cup	1.1
Tomato (raw)	1 small	1.5
Potato (boiled)	1 medium	2.0
Carrots (raw)	1 medium	2.3
Green beans (cooked)	¾ cup	3.2
Cauliflower (cooked)	1 cup	3.2
Brussels sprouts (cooked)	1 cup	4.5
Peas (cooked)	½ cup	6.2
Spinach (cooked)	½ cup	6.3
Kidney beans (cooked)	½ cup	7.4
Broccoli (cooked)	2 small stalks	11.5

Group V. Fats, Sweets, and Alcohol

These are foods we really need to be careful about. The only ones really necessary to life are the fats and oils, and we need only a modest amount—only eight to sixteen teaspoonfuls daily. Otherwise, the foods in this group contribute only calories, with at best a trace of nutrients easily obtained from other food groups at a lower cost in calories.

But fats, sweets, and alcohol provide something that can't be measured in calories or milligrams: *pleasure*. Most people really want some of these foods every day, and within the context of a balanced, varied, moderate diet, it's perfectly all right to enjoy your highballs and your hollandaise without adding to your cancer risk or to your hips.

Study the Trade-Offs carefully, adopt as many of the fat-saving strategies as you can, and you'll find it's not hard to achieve moderation without feeling shortchanged. Remember, the NAS committees does *not* recommend you eliminate these items from your way of life.

Fats

Though too much fat in your diet is dangerous, *some* fat is necessary to health. Without fats, the vitamins that can't dissolve in water (vitamins A, D, E, and K) can't be transported and made available throughout the body.

Fats are made up of units called fatty acids; these, in turn, are long chains of carbon atoms with hydrogen atoms bonded to them. The personality of the fat depends on whether the chain of carbon atoms carries as many hydrogen atoms as it can (saturated fat), has room for one or two more (monounsaturated fat), or can accept four or more additional hydrogen atoms (polyunsaturated fat).

Saturated fats are solid at room temperature; monounsaturated and polyunsaturated are liquid at room temperature and are commonly known as *oils*. To make polyunsaturated fats solid, manufacturers add hydrogen, converting some of the polyunsaturated fatty acids to saturated fatty acids. This process—*hydrogenation*—is what makes margarine spreadable. Hydrogenated shortenings and spreads are longer-lasting, more chemically stable, and less likely to spoil than are the oils from which they're made. Here is a list of the types of fats and their sources:

Type of Fat	Source	Examples
Polyunsaturated	Vegetable	Corn, cottonseed, safflower, sesame, soybean, sunflower oils
Monounsaturated	Vegetable	Olive oil, peanut oil
Saturated	Animal	Butter, lard, suet, meat drippings
	Vegetable	Coconut, palm oil
Hydrogenated	Vegetable with added hydrogen	Margarine, vegetable shortenings

167

Cooking Oils

With the NAS committee's suggestion that you divide your fat calories evenly between saturated fats (butter, lard, vegetable shortenings), polyunsaturated (corn, safflower, sesame, soybean, and sunflower oils), and monounsaturated (peanut and olive oils), you will use a variety of oils, instead of relying on just one. They all have different qualities—a half-and-half mixture of peanut oil and butter is the basis for much great cooking; the butter gives incomparable flavor and the peanut oil reduces the risk of burning. Peanut oil used alone is the best cooking oil I know of, and *the* indispensible oil for Oriental cooking. Sesame oil has a grand flavor all its own, so strong that you don't need much. I find I use it more for flavoring than for its merits as an oil. Polyunsaturated oils are good, all-around dependables, without much flavor. In marinades and salad dressings, you can substitute water for half the quantity of polyunsaturated oils and nobody will notice.

Butter. Don't stop using it altogether, just cut down. I've started keeping mine in the freezer, just to make me think twice before using it—and also because a quarter-pound now lasts me a long time. You can keep the good buttery taste in your cooking by using bland-tasting oils and adding a teaspoonful of butter.

Margarine. Use the polyunsaturated type—sparingly—if you must, but remember it's not a "free" food, it's *fat*! Try using other moist spreads like honey, apple butter, low-fat cottage cheese, on your toast instead.

Nuts and Seeds. They're high in fat, but also contain protease inhibitors, which inhibit carcinogenesis. Use some nuts and seeds in cooking now and then, where you can control the quantity, but don't eat them as "nibbles" with cocktails or as snacks—it's too easy to eat too many.

The assumption that all the fat in one's diet comes from meat or dairy products is quite wrong. Besides nuts and seeds, some foods that come from plants are abundant sources of fats—olives, avocados, nuts and coconuts in particular. We often add fat, unthinkingly, to low-fat foods. A simple green salad, slathered with dressing, may contain more fat than the good lean steak you eat with it. And research shows that people are not very good at identifying where fat comes from.

Baked goods, desserts of all kinds, sauces and gravies,

"made" dishes like stews and casseroles, fast foods, and mixes all tend to be high in fat, and we tend to believe that it's not there.

Furthermore, there's the untrimmable fat in processed meats. You can trim the fat from a pork chop but you can't take it out of a hot dog. The newer processed meats made from chicken or turkey, rather than beef or pork, are somewhat lower in fat than the traditional kinds, but they still contain more fat than plain poultry meat.

In planning your meals, cutting back on fat is going to require some thought. First of all, develop an awareness of where the fat in your present diet comes from—your *Brand-Name Nutrition Counter* will help you here, and the Department of Agriculture offers a fine booklet called *The Nutritive Value of Foods*. (Home and Garden Bulletin No. 72, available from Superintendent of Documents, U.S. Government Printing Office, Washington, D.C. 20402)

Next, decide the ways that you yourself would prefer to cut back. For me, one important step was to eat less cheese as a snack. I could have kept my cheese habit and brought my total fat calories into line by cutting way back on my fats from other sources—but that would have left me with a high proportion of saturated fat, compared to fat from other sources. The NAS recommends eating equal proportions of the three types of fats, so I chose to moderate my cheese addiction.

Finally, after deciding how to cut back on your fats, strive to vary the fats that you do eat from day to day. Allow yourself some spare ribs, hollandaise sauce, guacamole, and peanut butter—or whatever your favorite fatty foods may be. But don't indulge every day, and do it against a background of low-fat dairy products, lean meat, and prudent use of salad dressing.

Cholesterol

Authorities haven't yet agreed on how harmful dietary cholesterol really is. The body itself makes the 1,000 milligrams of cholesterol needed daily to aid in the production of vitamin D and certain hormones—this production decreases somewhat when a person takes in additional cholesterol in the diet, but not always enough to equal the amount eaten. People vary in the way they handle cholesterol, and in some, the level of cholesterol in the blood goes up when more cholesterol is added to the diet.

One thing is certain—nobody in nutrition advocates a high-cholesterol diet.

High cholesterol in the blood is thought by most experts to add to the risk of heart disease; and newly emerging evidence suggests that people who excrete cholesterol (in the form of bile acids) through the large intestine may run an increased risk of colon cancer.

But when we consider how to reduce the amount of cholesterol in the diet we run squarely into the fact that it's most highly concentrated in a very few of the most nutritious foods that we know—eggs and organ meats like liver and kidneys. Meats and milk contain much less, dissolved in the fat in milk and built into the cell walls of meat.

We can skim the fat from milk and eliminate much of its cholesterol content, but trimming the visible fat from meat doesn't affect the cholesterol in the lean parts.

Since lean meat is such a fine source of hard-to-get nutrients like zinc and other trace minerals, it makes sense to cut back on cholesterol contributed by other foods. Keeping down to three or four egg yolks a week and using low-fat dairy products routinely is the commonsense approach.

In addition, the less fat in your diet overall, the less efficiently your intestines can absorb the cholesterol you eat.

Sweets

These fall into two categories—intensely sweet foods which we use in small amounts to enhance the flavor of other foods, and items which contain high levels of sugar with other nutrients in fair amounts.

The most obvious example of the first type of sweet is plain granulated sugar—40 calories per tablespoonful with no other nutritive value whatsoever. In the same category are jams, jellies, syrups, honey, molasses, and candy. Though their calorie content varies, for our purposes we consider that a teaspoonful of one equals a teaspoonful of all the others. In the Everyday Food Plans, 7 to 18 teaspoonfuls of sugar and other sweets are permitted daily, but if you can live with less, you can spend those calories on foods that provide more nutrients—such as fresh fruits.

The second type of sweet food is the whole assortment of desserts, pastries, cakes, cookies, puddings, frozen treats, and so forth. These contain sugar, in substantial quantity, and various ingredients from other food groups, such as fats, milk and milk products, flour and grains, and fruits. Because of the mixture of ingredients, it's hard to determine where a food like a piece of cake fits into your daily scheme of things. This is where the Trade-Offs can really help—a slice of white cake with chocolate icing counts as one slice of bread plus 6 tablespoons of sugar plus 3 teaspoons of fat.

Except insofar as they add to your daily total of calories, which in turn can lead to obesity which adds to your cancer risk, the NAS committee finds no direct link between sugar and cancer. That's why, when you're having your toast or bagel in the morning, you'd be much better off spreading it with a teaspoonful of honey or jam than a teaspoonful of butter or margarine. It's *fat* that directly heightens cancer risk, and while sugar *in excess* is not good for you, small amounts have a place in a balanced, varied, moderate diet, and can help you cut down on your fat intake.

Artificial Sweeteners

The NAS committee did not find that saccharin poses enough of a risk of cancer to humans to warrant any words of warning. Saccharin seems to be at most a weak promoter in animals; whether this is true in human beings is questionable since, in the eighty-plus years it's been in wide use, no consistent increase in cancer among saccharin users has been seen.

As a sugar substitute, however, saccharin has some drawbacks. Many people find it has an objectionable bitter aftertaste. Furthermore, neither saccharin nor the recently introduced aspartame, another noncaloric sugar substitute (the chemical name for the artificial sweetener marketed as Nutra-Sweet or Equal), can provide the proper texture to baked goods like cakes or cookies, and cannot be used to make traditional kinds of sugar candies.

Saccharin in coffee or tea probably poses no serious threat to your health, provided you drink only a few cups daily. In view of its possible role as a promoter, albeit a weak one, prudence suggests that we take a rest from saccharin periodically, going back to sugar in our coffee for a week or two and adjusting our sugar consumption elsewhere to make up for it.

It's not a good idea to allow children to develop a lifelong habit of drinking saccharin-free soft drinks—or for adults to imbibe half a dozen cans every day. Explore other possibilities (what ever happened to the jug of plain water that every family used to keep in the refrigerator?).

One way to wean children from the diet-soda habit is to get them interested in concocting their own "cocktails" of fruit juices—fresh, bottled, or from frozen concentrate.

A great big covered container of cranberry-apple-orange juice, diluted for economy with water or seltzer, is fun to keep in the refrigerator. Cider, heated up with a sprinkle of spices, is a warming after-school treat; did you know you can serve cranberry juice the same way?

Similarly, convenient cans of cold diet soda at a picnic add no cancer risk so long as you don't have a picnic every day.

Alcohol

No one suggests that a return to Prohibition would be a workable approach to the role that heavy drinking plays in the development of some kinds of cancer, but in view of the evidence it's just common sense to review the place of alcohol in our lives. Alcohol contributes empty calories to the diet, and if you want a couple of glasses of wine with your dinner or a cold beer on a hot afternoon, you must allow for these calories by adjusting your consumption of other foods.

For practical purposes, though it's not biochemically accurate, we can gauge the calorie-effect of alcohol in terms of sugar: a can of beer equals 10 teaspoons of sugar, a glass of dry white wine equals 6, and other alcoholic beverages, as the Trade-Offs indicate, have intermediate amounts of calories.

"If you drink alcohol, do it in moderation," says the NAS committee. Their definition of moderation is one or two drinks daily as a general rule, though an *occasional* celebration with larger amounts probably does not increase cancer risk for otherwise light-to-moderate drinkers.

Except for vodka and very light colored liquors, most forms of alcohol contain congeners—some of which are cancer promoters. Danger could arise from drinking large quantities of the same kind of liquor, year after year. Common sense would dictate, then, that we *vary* our alcoholic beverages, just as we vary our foods, particularly if we tend to drink more than a glass or two each day.

A Word about Sodium

The NAS committee found the epidemiological evidence linking heavily salt-cured, salt-pickled, and smoked foods (which are often heavily salted, too) with cancer of the stomach so telling that they issued a specific warning against eating large quantities of these foods.

There is no similarly clear-cut evidence associating lower levels of sodium with cancer.

But we do know that other problems can arise from taking in more than the 200 milligrams of sodium a person really requires each day. The most annoying and apparent symptom is fluid retention, which can make you feel bloated and too big for your clothes, and which can give your face a puffy appearance. That's bad enough, but the insidious, less apparent result of too much sodium is *hypertension*, or high blood pressure.

Hypertension has no symptoms; the only way to know whether you have it is to have your blood pressure checked. Hypertension can lead to heart disease, the number-one killer in the U.S., to stroke, and to other cardiovascular problems. The patient who is diagnosed with cancer and who has any of these problems on top of the malignancy is in very serious trouble, for these underlying conditions can complicate the treatment of cancer enormously.

The sodium in our diet gets there in two ways—from added salty tasting ingredients (table salt, baking soda, baking powder, sodium nitrite and sodium nitrate used as preservatives, and monosodium glutamate), and from the foods themselves. Regular milk contains around 125 milligrams of sodium per cup; low-fat milk with added dry solids has slightly more. Natural cheese has 75 to 300 milligrams of sodium per ounce; processed cheeses have 350 to 450 milligrams. Half a cup of low-fat cottage cheese contains about 450 milligrams of sodium. Dried peas and beans are high in sodium, with 800 to 1,300 milligrams per cup serving. Meats, fish, eggs, and poultry contain some sodium, usually less than 75 milligrams per three-ounce serving. Grains, and fresh and frozen fruits and vegetables are low in sodium.

Sodium sneaks in when foods are processed, packaged, and prepared. The more manipulations a food has gone through, the more opportunities there have been for the marketers to throw in salt and other sodium compounds, probably to give the consumer the idea that there is more going on in terms of flavor than there might otherwise seem.

Cured meats like ham, bologna, hot dogs, and the like have 750 to 1,350 milligrams of sodium per three-ounce serving. Frozen or canned meat dishes, like pasta with beef, lasagna, ravioli, potpies, and the like have from 850 to 1,400 milligrams of sodium for every cup (8 ounces). Canned vegetables are quite high in sodium, and so are those handy frozen vegetables-in-a-sauce; these can contain 250 to 450 milligrams of sodium per half-cup serving.

White or whole-grain breads contain between 110 and 150 milligrams of sodium per slice. Oatmeal and other hot cereals have 5 milligrams or less in a half-cup serving—unless you add salt yourself. Cold cereals vary in their sodium content; some have little or no added sodium, but you have to read the label to find which they are.

Some foods are *meant* to be salty—potato chips, salted nuts, and crispy munching snacks generally have 150 to 300 milligrams of sodium per ounce; pretzels and salted popcorn have even more. The saltiness is part of the personality of these foods.

And then there are piquant extras that we pour, shake, and sprinkle over other foods which may themselves be low in sodium. Soy sauce has 1,000 milligrams of sodium per tablespoon; Worcestershire sauce, mustard, ketchup, chili sauce, and such have about 125 to 127 milligrams per tablespoon. Bottled salad dressings have 100 to 250 milligrams of sodium per tablespoon.

Taking in more than 200 milligrams of sodium daily won't hurt you if you keep levels low. The NAS Food and Nutrition Board says that 1,100 to 3,300 milligrams daily is safe and adequate. That is equivalent to 3 to 8 grams of salt. But most of us average between 2,300 and 6,900 milligrams daily, and many eat more.

If you are interested in avoiding cancer, you are, I hope,

interested in maintaining good health generally, and that ought to include a low-sodium approach to food. Here are some pointers—if you'd like more, get a copy of *Sodium: Think About It* (U.S. Department of Agriculture and U.S. Department of Health and Human Services, Home and Garden Bulletin No. 237).

- Cook as many foods "from scratch" as you can. Processed foods, "convenience" foods, and mixes tend to contain extra sodium. When you're the cook, you're in charge.
- Don't add salt during cooking. (Besides adding sodium, it tends to make foods mushy in texture.) Correct the seasoning just before you serve.
- Use products like low-sodium ketchup, soy sauce, and salad dressing, or better still, make your own and leave out the salt.
- Be clever with other seasonings and you won't need so much salt. Lemon juice, pepper, vinegar, spices, and herbs may make salt unnecessary in some recipes. It really depends on the food, however—you can't just sprinkle curry powder on everything and expect your family not to notice you've made a drastic change in your cuisine.
- Don't try to eliminate salt entirely all at once. Your taste for salt was *acquired*, and can be unlearned gradually.
- Plan your meals intelligently. If you're serving ham, surround it with low-salt foods like coleslaw in a low-sodium dressing, vegetables in a curry sauce made without salt, and lots of fresh fruit. Save the pickles and potato chips for a meal otherwise low in sodium.
- Don't look for shortcuts. Salt substitutes generally contain potassium compounds, which can aggravate kidney problems or interfere with medications a person may be taking. If you're on a medication that slows potassium excretion, a high-potassium salt substitute can lead to a high concentration of potassium in the body that can cause heart trouble. Try sodium-eliminating strategies first, and consider salt substitutes as a last resort, clearing them first with your doctor.

- And don't pay extra money for sea salt, thinking it will help you solve the sodium problem. It's still just plain sodium chloride, with a *slight* amount of trace minerals, too little to make any difference unless you use more of the salt than is good for you.
- My mother, who has more character than anyone else in the world, cut down on sodium by disciplining herself not to put salt on her morning sunny-side up egg. She figured that since that was the food that seemed to her to need salt most of all, eliminating salt from her egg would make everything else easy.

18

The Everyday Food Plans

How Many Calories Do You Need?

The Recommended Daily Calorie Intake tables from the Food and Nutrition Board of the National Academy of Sciences are a rough guide to how many calories a person needs. (See Tables 3 and 4.)

Please note that the calorie levels are given as a *range*—

Table 3

Suggested Desirable Weights for Heights and Ranges for Adult Males and Females

Height (Inches)	Men Weight (Range)	Women Weight (Range)
58		102 (92–119)
60		107 (96–125)
62	123 (112–141)	113 (102–131)
64	130 (118–148)	120 (108–138)
66	136 (124–156)	128 (114–146)
68	145 (132–166)	136 (122–154)
70	154 (140–174)	144 (130–163)
72	162 (148–184)	152 (138–173)
74	171 (156–194)	
76	181 (164–204)	

Source: Recommended Daily Allowances, National Academy of Sciences, Food and Nutrition Board, 1980.

specific calorie intakes for people of specific age, height, and weight are provided, but that's just to give a ball-park idea. For instance, a fifty-year-old man, 5 feet 8 inches tall and weighing 154 pounds, is allowed 2,700 calories daily. But if he's larger in stature, or leads a very active life, he should have more calories—up to 3,100. Similarly, a twenty-three-year-old woman, 5 feet 4 inches tall and weighing 120 pounds, is, according to the table, permitted 2,000 calories. If her life is sedentary, she should probably gear her eating to the lower end of the range—closer to 1,600 calories.

And as age increases, a person's calorie intake should move along with it. The 3,300 calories required by an active

Table 4

Recommended Daily Calorie Intake for Mean Age and Height

	Age (Years)	Weight (Lbs.)	Height (Inches)	Calories (Range)
Children	1–3	29	35	1,300 (900–1,800)
	4–6	44	44	1,700 (1,300–2,300)
	7–10	62	52	2,400 (1,650–3,300)
Males	11–14	99	62	2,700 (2,000–3,700)
	15–18	145	69	2,800 (2,100–3,900)
	19–22	154	70	2,900 (2,700–3,900)
	23–50	154	70	2,700 (2,300–3,100)
	51–75	154	70	2,400 (2,000–2,800)
	70+	154	70	2,050 (1,650–2,450)
Females	11–14	101	62	2,200 (1,500–3,000)
	15–18	120	64	2,100 (1,200–3,000)
	19–22	120	64	2,100 (1,700–2,500)
	23–50	120	64	2,000 (1,600–2,400)
	51–75	120	64	1,800 (1,400–2,200)
	76+	120	64	1,600 (1,200–2,000)
Pregnancy				add 300
Lactation				add 500

Source: Recommended Daily Allowances, National Academy of Sciences, Food and Nutrition Board, 1980.

en-year-old aren't enough to keep a college athlete going—3,900 daily calories are necessary for a young man who runs seriously or performs heavy manual labor.

How many calories do you really need? Your best guide is your own body. If you're healthy, neither too fat nor too thin, and if your appetite is good, you are probably eating the appropriate number of calories. (If you want to gain or lose weight, see Special Strategies for Special People, page 189.)

But taking in the proper number of calories daily is only part of healthy eating. As we've noted, those calories must be spent wisely to get the maximum good nutrition from the foods you eat. And your diet should be planned intelligently enough to permit you a reasonable amount of the sweet, fatty, and alcoholic items that you *enjoy*, but which mustn't be the backbone of your daily food plan.

The U.S. Department of Agriculture eating patterns take these objectives into account, and Everyday Food Plans is based on their carefully formulated diet.

These plans are designed to provide, over the course of a week, the nutrients you need, within the calorie range that you require, with a reasonable amount of fat, sugar, and alcohol (if you want it) for fun. They are not intended to be rigid, and the Trade-Off system allows you to be extremely flexible in your choices. That flexibility will insure the kind of balanced, varied, and moderate diet that will help you reduce your risk of cancer in future years, and maintain good health here and now.

These eating plans are intended to guide you gently into the habit of eating some foods from each of the *basic four food groups* every day. The four groups—milk, milk products, and cheese; meat, fish, and poultry; fruits and vegetables; and breads, grains, and cereals—are all broad enough for everybody to find a number of appealing foods to choose from every day. If you don't like milk, you can use the Trade-Offs to obtain your milk benefits from cheese, yogurt, ice cream, and other foods in the dairy group. If you have a strong prejudice in favor of red meat (beef and lamb)—or against it, for that matter—you can concentrate on the meat-group foods that you particularly like.

But if you've read the earlier chapters of this book carefully, I hope that you will see the benefits in *not* sticking with the same types of food. People who shun red meat are passing up a superb source of protein, phosphorus, iron, and zinc, plus vitamins B_6 and B_{12}—which are found in few other foods. People who never eat fish or shellfish miss out on a grand array of trace minerals. People who exclude completely a particular food may not be getting some extremely important constituent—perhaps one that hasn't even been discovered yet.

Naturally, people who are eating at the higher end of the calorie range have a lot more flexibility in their diet. At 2,800 calories, four daily servings of vegetables are permitted, meaning that a person can choose a half-cup serving of dark-green vegetables, a half cup of deep-yellow vegetables, a half cup of starchy vegetable, and a half cup of another type—an artichoke, perhaps, or cauliflower. No need to worry about consuming all the vitamin A, vitamin C, beta-carotene, indoles, flavones, fiber, and other good things you need when you have lots of calories to work with.

But if you have only 1,600 calories to spend on nutrition every day, then the vegetables are limited to *two* servings. It's impossible to touch all the bases every day at that calorie level, so *weekly* planning becomes important. Switching choices around among the dark-green, deep-yellow, and cruciferae enables us to take in, over the course of a week, a good assortment of vegetables and a wide array of nutrients. On days when I don't eat a deep-yellow vegetable such as carrots or pumpkin, I make sure to eat a deep-yellow *fruit*, like cantaloupe, apricots, or papaya (a half cup of cut-up papaya equals 1,225 international units of vitamin A!).

Once you have established eating habits based on these patterns—and it isn't difficult at all—you can allow yourself to stray, now and then. Nobody is going to arrest you for eating a steak or a slab of chocolate cake, and if you splurge occasionally, the balanced, varied, moderate nutritional foundation that you've already laid for yourself will protect you. But indulge *wisely*—prepare for a luxurious meal by cutting back on the size of your servings, or by eating a few meals particularly low in fat and high in fiber, over the course of a few days. And go lightly for a day or so afterward.

In order to help you spread your nutrition sensibly throughout the day, the Everyday Food Plans suggest that you have this many servings of grain foods for breakfast, that many servings of vegetables at lunch, and so forth, but you may not want to follow these patterns every day. Maybe you'd rather have an egg for breakfast. In that case, of course, subtract one ounce of meat, fish, or poultry from one of your other meals. If you'd prefer a slice of cake for dessert at dinnertime, you can save up some slices of bread from other meals and combine them with fat and sugar from your daily allowances (see Trade-Offs).

And you can, of course, save up equivalents of meat, grains, fats, and sugar from day to day in anticipation of a special meal, or skip your nightly drink during the week when a couple of weekend parties are coming up, but remember to eat *some* food from *each* group every day.

You Don't Have to Count Calories!

Going through a lot of arithmetic to find the number of calories in a portion of food, and to decide how much of one you can substitute for another, is largely a waste of time.

Our foods, after all, are derived from plants and animals, and since living things vary, the nutritional content of separate but identical servings of the same food can vary, too.

Since your daily diet is not a scientific experiment, in which every nutrient must be measured and accounted for, you can get a good enough idea of the calories and other nutrients you're ingesting from the approximate values in *The Brand Name Nutrition Counter* and *The Nutritive Value of Foods*. If you're five calories off on one food, it will almost certainly be balanced by another small inaccuracy elsewhere.

Modern nutritionists have decided that it makes more sense to measure nutritional value, including calories, in terms of how much of a food within one of the four main groups is equivalent to another food within the same group. The term they use is Trade-Off.

Trade-Offs aren't precisely equivalent to each other. Half a 3-inch bagel contains 82.5 calories, a slice of pumpernickel 5 by 4 by ⅜ inches has 80 calories, and a slice of soft white enriched bread (18 slices to the loaf) contains 70 calories. Yet the U.S. Department of Agriculture says we can count them as equivalent to each other.

Although half a cup of cooked carrots is not nutritionally

Vegetables		Fats	Sugar	Alcohol
Vary your choices; favor deep yellow, dark green, & cruciferae		Aim for equal amounts of saturated, mono-unsaturated, polyunsaturated. Be sure to include nuts & seeds	Including honey, syrup, & molasses	If you drink, deduct from your sugar allowance See Trade-Offs
½ cup =	1 cup raw, leafy vegetables	1 teaspoon (8–16 teaspoons daily)	1 teaspoon (7–18 teaspoons)	1–2 drinks daily limit
1	2	8	7	See above
	2	2	2	
	1	2	2	
1	1	2	2	
		2	1	
1	2	10	9	See above
	2	3	2	
	1	3	3	
1	1	3	2	
		2	2	
1	3	13	16	See above
	3	3	4	
	1	3	4	
	2	3	4	
		4	4	
2	4	16	18	See above
	3	3	4	
1	2	3	4	
1	2	5	5	
		5	5	

identical to half a cup of cooked broccoli, this system uses them interchangeably. Within the vegetable group, we assume that one vegetable is equal to another (providing we limit the starchy ones like corn, peas, dried beans to one to two servings daily).

Please note, however, that the Trade-Offs can be made only *within* a food group. You can't drink a cup of low-fat milk and count it as the equivalent of two half-cup servings of vegetables. And though the Trade-Off system assumes that lean meat, skinned chicken, and fish are equivalent, ounce for ounce, to each other, they are not equivalent to the same amount of fruit. The system cleverly forces us to eat some foods from each group every day.

Within prescribed limits, certain substitutions from one group to another are permitted, however.

Let's say you want a piece of old-fashioned fried chicken—knowing, of course, that its crispy breaded coating has absorbed some fat during the cooking process. How does that fit into a day's good eating?

The Trade-Offs on page 186 tell us that half a breast of chicken, deep-fried in batter, counts as half a breast of chicken, roasted, plus 1 slice of bread, plus 2 teaspoons of fat. Go ahead and eat your fried chicken, and enjoy it, subtracting one slice of bread from your day's grain allowance, and two teaspoons of fat from the fat allotment.

Similarly, a cup of cooked lentils (or other dried peas or beans) dressed with a teaspoonful of olive oil (plus lemon juice, chopped onion and parsley, with mint and pepper flakes for piquancy) can stand in for a sandwich made with two ounces of meat on two slices of bread. And vice-versa, of course.

The Trade-Offs work only when you deal with the foods in terms of standard serving size: half a cup of fruit or vegetables, a slice of bread or half a cup of cooked grain products, a cup of milk, and ounce-for-ounce amounts of meat, fish, and poultry. You may eat more of these foods in a meal, however, so you must remember to think of the *number of standard servings* you eat. If you eat a full cup of coleslaw, that would count as two half-cup servings.

The USDA puts eggs in the meat-fish-poultry group, which means that for our purposes, a whole egg equals an ounce of any of these foods. Because of egg yolks' high cholesterol content, people really shouldn't consume more than three or four egg yolks per week. The good news is that you can have as many egg *whites* as you want. (They're only 15 calories each.) Depending on the size of the eggs, you can make the equivalent of a two-egg omelette or serving of scrambled eggs from one whole egg plus one (or more) egg whites.

Use the Trade-Offs in the light of what research has told us about the value of a balanced, varied, moderate diet. Don't stick with the same foods day after day. Vary your choices within each food group—the Trade-Offs make it easy—and aim for as wide a range of foods as their availability and your pocketbook allow.

The Trade-Offs

I. *The Dairy Group*
Milk, cheeses, and yogurt. A serving is one cup of whole milk or its equivalent.

1 cup whole milk	= 1 cup skim milk + 2 teaspoons fat
1 cup 2% fat milk	= 1 cup skim milk + 1 teaspoon fat
1 cup 2% fat chocolate milk	= 1 cup skim milk + 1 teaspoon fat + 3 teaspoons sugar
8 oz. plain low-fat yogurt	= 1 cup skim milk + 1 teaspoon fat
8 oz. low-fat vanilla yogurt	= 1 cup skim milk + 1 teaspoon fat + 4 teaspoons sugar
8 oz. low-fat fruit yogurt	= 1 cup skim milk + 1 teaspoon fat + 7 teaspoons sugar
1½ oz. natural cheese	= 1 cup skim milk + 3 teaspoons fat
2 oz. processed American cheese	= 1 cup skim milk + 4 teaspoons fat

II. *The Grain Group*
Cereals, breads, and grains. A serving is one slice of bread.

1 slice	bread	= 4 small crackers (2 large)
1 slice	bread	= ½ cup *cooked* pasta, rice, or cereal
1 slice	bread	= ½ English muffin, ½ hamburger roll, ½ bagel, ½ large dinner roll

1	slice	bread	= 1 ounce ready-to-eat cereal (don't try to measure by volume, since the same weight of cereal will occupy different space in the cup depending on size and shape of flakes)
1	slice	bread	= 1 small roll, muffin, or biscuit

Note: At least half the servings from this group should come from products made of *whole grains*—but count whole-grain products as equivalent to those made from white enriched flour.

III. *The Meat Group*

Meat, fish, poultry, and eggs. A serving is 2 to 4 ounces of meat, fish, or poultry, with visible fat removed before cooking. Chicken, turkey, and fish should be skinned.

1 whole egg	= 1 ounce of meat, fish, or poultry	
2 oz. bologna, luncheon meat, or hot dog	= 1 ounce lean meat, fish, or poultry	+ 3 ounces fat
½ chicken breast, deep-fried with batter coating	= ½ chicken breast roasted	+ 1 slice white bread + 2 teaspoons fat
½ cup cooked dried beans or peas	= 1 oz. lean meat, fish, or poultry	+ 1 teaspoon fat + 1 slice bread
2 tablespoons peanut butter	= 1 oz. lean meat, fish, or poultry	+ 3 teaspoons fat
¼ cup seeds	= 1 oz. lean meat, fish, or poultry	+ 4 teaspoons fat
⅓ cup nuts	= 1 oz. lean meat, fish, or poultry	+ 5 teaspoons fat

IV. *The Vegetable and Fruit Group*

Vegetables. A serving is ½ cup.

½ cup solid vegetables	= 1 cup raw, leafy vegetables	
10 french fries	= 1 medium boiled potato	+ 2 teaspoons fat

It's important to vary your choices, and except for the starchy vegetables (which contain valuable nutrients but which should be limited to a serving or two daily), you can interchange vegetables freely. Dried peas and beans are more heavily loaded with nutrients than other vegetables, and because of their protein content they can serve as a substitute for meat, fish, or poultry (see above).

Fruits. A serving equals an average-sized piece of whole fruit, 6 ounces of fruit juice, ½ cup of berries or sliced or cooked fruit, or ¼ cup of dried fruit.

½ cup frozen sweetened fruit	= ½ cup fresh or frozen fruit (unsweetened)	+ 6 teaspoons sugar
½ cup fruit canned in light syrup	= ½ cup unsweetened fruit	+ 2 teaspoons sugar
½ cup canned fruit in heavy syrup	= ½ cup unsweetened fruit	+ 4 teaspoons sugar

The Extras.

Fats, sweets, and alcohol. Handle with care. All are concentrated sources of calories and easy to lose track of in the daily diet.

Fats shouldn't exceed 8 to 16 teaspoons daily, including what you eat in baked goods, soups, stews, and the like; the exact level depends on your proper calorie intake.

1 teaspoon margarine, butter, or oil	= 5 teaspoons sour cream
1 teaspoon margarine, butter, or oil	= 4 teaspoons light cream
3 teaspoons cream cheese	= 1 teaspoon margarine, butter, or oil
2 teaspoons bottled Italian salad dressing	= 1 teaspoon margarine, butter, or oil

Sugar is sugar, whether it's white or brown, crystal in form or syrupy. All candy, syrups (corn, maple, molasses, honey), jams and jellies, and sweet desserts (including ices and sherbets as well as the frosting on a cake) count the same as sugar from the sugar bowl.

1 teaspoon jam, jelly, or marmalade	= 1 teaspoon sugar, honey, or molasses
12 oz. sugar-sweetened cola drink	= 9 teaspoons sugar
12 oz. canned or bottled fruit drink, punch, or ade (noncarbonated)	= 12 teaspoons sugar
1 ounce chocolate bar = 5 teaspoons sugar + 2 teaspoons fat	

At 1,600 calories daily, your sugar intake shouldn't exceed 7 teaspoons per day; at the 2,800-calorie level, you can have up to 18 teaspoons sugar.

Alcohol. It's really metabolized somewhat like a fat, but it's easier to visualize its caloric equivalents when you compare alcoholic beverages to sugar.

12 oz. beer	= 10 teaspoons sugar
3½ oz. wine (white or red)	= 6 teaspoons sugar
3½ oz. sweet dessert wine	= 9 teaspoons sugar
1½ oz. whiskey, vodka, gin, rum	= 7 teaspoons sugar

Trade-Offs for calorie-dense treats. Some of these foods contain good nutrients, and can't be considered empty calories in the strict sense, but along with the protein, vitamins, and minerals comes more fat than you're likely to need.

18 potato chips	= 1 medium boiled potato	+ 3 teaspoons fat
1 medium slice apple pie	= 2 slices bread	+ ⅓ medium apple + 6 teaspoons sugar + 3 teaspoons fat
1 small slice white cake with chocolate frosting	= 1 slice bread	+ 6 teaspoons sugar + 3 teaspoons fat
2 oatmeal cookies	= 1 slice bread	+ 1 teaspoon sugar + 1 teaspoon fat
½ cup low-fat frozen yogurt	= ⅓ cup skim milk	+ 4 teaspoons sugar
½ cup ice milk	= ⅓ cup skim milk	+ 3 teaspoons sugar + 1 teaspoon fat

½ cup ice cream   = ⅓ cup skim milk + 3 teaspoons sugar
                                          + 2 teaspoons fat

Special Strategies for Special People

The NAS guidelines, and the principles of balanced, varied, moderate nutrition, are applicable to everybody—young and old, athlete and TV addict. But for some people, putting these principles to work requires a little extra thought and planning, and for specific groups (smokers, teenagers, people who need to lose or gain weight) there are special dietary needs.

In this section, you'll find some practical suggestions for meeting the out-of-the-ordinary requirements of people of different ages and life-styles.

Feeding the Children

Parents have two kinds of responsibilities in feeding their children—to see that they're properly nourished now, and to impart good eating habits and attitudes to last a lifetime. The foods a child learns to like can have important effects on his or her cancer risks.

Obviously, children need enough calories and nutrients to stay healthy and grow properly. Most children have no problem getting enough calories; more often difficulties lie in preventing obesity and in ensuring that the calories bring in the right assortment of nutrients.

By example, more than by preaching, parents educate their children, for good or ill, about food, whether it's intentional or not. Just as a too-sugary childhood diet can lead to dental problems that may plague a person for a lifetime, ideas about food acquired early in life can affect one's health for years to come. A home where rich desserts are offered as rewards, where salads are regarded as "sissy," and steak must be burned beyond recognition teaches children to make choices that add up to increased cancer risks in later life.

If some foods aren't served at home, children are likely to reject them later. If Daddy won't eat lamb, or if the family won't touch cabbage, children will absorb these lessons and resist trying those foods. Parents who indulge in low-nutrition snacks or make alcoholic beverages a large part of their lives are setting nutritional examples that children are likely to imitate later on. It won't help to insist that these foods are "for grownups"—kids aren't fooled by double standards.

But it can work the other way. Parents can show by their own eating behavior that a balanced, varied, moderate diet is desirable and fun. You can scarcely teach a child good eating habits by giving him or her a handful of carrot sticks while *you* wolf down the donuts.

Some points for parents to remember:

- Children's stomachs are small. Though regular mealtimes are important, there should be regular snacktimes (at midmorning and midafternoon) to prevent small children from becoming so tired and hungry that they lose their appetites. Young appetites are best early in the day.
- Children need to be encouraged to eat a variety of foods. Instead of letting them eat unlimited quantities of their favorites, give them *small* servings of *many* foods.
- Watch out for milk. It can easily become a junk food, since children may drink so much of it they have no room for anything else. A child who drinks four to five cups of milk a day gets unnecessary calories and no additional nutritional benefits, since milk is low in iron and vitamin C. After a child is one year old, two cups of milk each day provide almost seventy-five percent of his daily calcium needs. The commonsense solution is to serve small amounts of milk throughout the day, with whole-grain crackers for snacks.
- Chewing is hard work for baby teeth. The molar teeth that grind foods don't appear till a child is six or so; until then, it's hard to cope with tough, dry foods. That's why hamburgers and frankfurters are more popular with preschoolers than hard-to-chew steak. Crunchy, fiber-rich foods like carrots and other raw vegetables may be difficult for small children to chew; nevertheless, they should be introduced early. (A cold carrot is a soothing treat for a teething baby, and introduces the idea of raw vegetables as snacks.) As a child learns to chew better, increase the crisp and crunchy foods—don't let children get used to a soft diet.
- Extremes in flavor and temperature don't appeal to small children. While some children adore pizza and pickles

(probably because they see the rest of the family enjoying them often), most resist unfamiliar, strongly flavored foods. They also seem to prefer food served at room temperature, rather than icy cold or piping hot. (How often have you watched a toddler stir his ice cream until it's the temperature of warm milk?) Keep these facts in mind when introducing a new food to your family. Go lightly on exotic seasonings for the younger members, and don't insist that they try a new food when it's extremely hot or cold.

- Don't go overboard with fruit juices. Orange juice contains about the same number of calories, ounce for ounce, as regular soft drinks. The only advantage is that juice also contains vitamin C, folic acid, thiamine, and potassium, whereas the soda offers mere empty calories. Juices should be drunk in moderation and if you think your children are overdoing them, dilute the juice with water. Forget about "fruit punch" and canned or bottled "fruit drinks"—they've been pumped full of vitamin C (available in regular foods) but otherwise contain nothing much except sugar.

- Children *can* enjoy vegetables. A good parental example helps, of course, but good preparation goes a surprisingly long way. Overcooked vegetables are mushy in texture, unattractive in color, and may smell or taste unpleasant—in other words, they're "yucky" for both children and adults. Preserve the good taste and fresh looks of vegetables by microwaving, steaming, or stir-frying them; if you boil them, leave the cover off the pot and the color will be better. Cruciferae should be cooked in open pots with plenty of water to keep the odor to a minimum.

- Think up clever and attractive ways to serve vegetables, and encourage your children to help prepare them. They can use cookie cutters to cut fancy shapes from carrots, red or green peppers, or zucchini slices; picture a handful of bright-colored stars cut from slices of large carrot, added to a dish of chopped broccoli, and sweet red-pepper hearts decorating cauliflower for Valentine's Day. Children are fascinated with grated, shredded, and minced vegetables; the older ones can use grinders and graters to make a heap of shredded beets or carrots to sprinkle on other foods.

191

- The transition to healthier snacks and treats can be eased by encouraging the children to make their own. Instead of ice cream, try popsicles made from plain yogurt and fresh fruit, frozen in your own freezer; experiment with variations using raisins, nuts, granola. Bake your own cookies, and let the children help. Those who are too young to use sharp cookie cutters can use an inverted plastic cup and decorate the cookies with raisins, cut-up dried fruit, and so forth. Instead of packaged high-calorie treats, sweet "sandwiches" can be made from slices of fresh fruit filled with low-fat ricotta cheese (flavored with vanilla, lemon or orange peel, cinnamon) or dried apricots or prunes puréed in a food processor. Preteens may enjoy raw vegetables served with a yogurt or peanut-butter dip.

Teenagers

Adolescence is a time of strikingly rapid growth, when boys typically double their weight and grow about 13½ inches in height, while girls grow about 9 inches and gain about 49 pounds. During this time, teenagers need a variety of foods to provide the wide range of nutrients their bodies require.

A balanced, varied, moderate diet like that described for adults in this book will keep a teenager from becoming deficient in vitamin A. Don't forget that vitamin A supplements, especially when taken over a long time, can cause dangerous toxicity to the skin and nervous system. Teenagers who consider themselves "into nutrition" should stay away from vitamin A supplements and concentrate on getting this vitamin from whole foods.

Teenage eating patterns may lead to vitamin C deficiency. Skipping breakfast and the orange juice or grapefruit that's a traditional part of the meal may be one reason. Another is the tendency of teens to snack on low-vitamin C fast foods, instead of fruit or raw vegetables. Just one serving of citrus fruits, strawberries, cantaloupes, or a high-vitamin C vegetable like cabbage or tomatoes, is enough to meet a teenager's need for this crucial vitamin.

For the extra calcium they need, teenagers should have an extra serving of milk or milk products every day—that's a total of three servings daily. If weight is a problem, dairy products should be low-fat.

Teens with low calorie intakes, or those whose nutrition is otherwise unbalanced might need an iron supplement. Ask your doctor about this.

Calorie needs among teenagers vary tremendously, depending on their level of physical activity. A boy on the varsity football team may need 4,000 to 6,000 calories daily; a studious girl may need only 2,000. Your teenager is getting enough calories when he or she has a healthy appetite and is in a weight range appropriate for height and body size.

Teenagers often worry about their appearance—indeed, it may seem to be an obsession. They frequently go on reducing diets or decide to become vegetarians, and if an unbalanced fad diet or severely limited calorie intake becomes a way of life for too long, it may slow a young person's rate of growth.

But if a teenager is within the normal weight range and is simply experimenting with a fad diet or a vegetarian regime, a parent can probably be most helpful by simply providing good information, offering a variety of healthy foods, and meddling as little as possible. Here are some tips on guiding teenage nutrition:

- Encourage overweight teenagers to increase physical activity. Serve as a good role model yourself, maintaining your own proper weight through good eating habits and exercise. Keep empty-calorie snacks and rich foods out of the pantry and refrigerator. But remember that the responsibility for losing or gaining weight lies with your son or daughter, not with you.
- Peer pressure, religious principles, or expected health benefits may inspire adolescents to become vegetarians. If their regime is of the *lacto-ovo* vegetarian kind, they will be able to get most of the nutrients they need from the food they eat, but the strict vegetarian diet (*vegan*) which excludes all animal products is inadequate in the vitamin B_{12}, iron, calcium, riboflavin, and vitamin D that a growing teenager requires.
- Teach your teenagers to *cook*! This will make them feel more adult and independent and may encourage an inter-

est in good nutrition. Let them experiment with new recipes. Information about his or her daily food requirements can come from casual discussions or from cookbooks, reference guides, USDA pamphlets. Ask teenagers to cook a family dinner once in a while.

- Make it easy for teenagers to snack healthily. Stock the kitchen with: ready-to-eat cold cereals that aren't high in sugar; homemade batter for whole-grain pancakes, waffles, and french toast; fresh and dried fruits; milk, yogurt, cheese, cottage cheese; whole-grain breads, and crackers; fresh vegetables suitable for snacking (carrots, green peppers, tomatoes).

- Make extra low-fat main-dish foods for dinner so the remainder can be stored in the refrigerator. Teenagers love to snack on leftovers.

- Note when your teenager is likely to be especially hungry, and make sure the kitchen is replete with nutritious snacks and the makings for informal meals. These times might be: after soccer practice; during exam time; after choir rehearsal; when friends sleep over . . .

- Set a good example. If the parents skip meals, fool around with fad diets, experience dramatic gains and losses in weight, and repeat every rumor about cancer threats or miracle cures from foods, you can hardly expect a young person in the family not to follow suit. As you change your own eating habits to achieve a more balanced, varied, and moderate diet, your teenagers may very well adopt a saner eating style themselves—without a nagging word from you!

Teenagers probably aren't likely to pay much attention to the message that poor eating habits now may add to their risk of cancer later on. The best that a parent can do is to make sure that there are plenty of low-fat snacks around. Someday, a teenager may become interested in nutrition, either in hopes of losing or gaining weight, or because of a general interest in health. At that time, he or she may become even more enthusiastic about an anticancer life-style than you are.

Low-Fat Snacks
(Especially for Teenagers)

Angel food cake

Frozen cubes of fruit juice

Hot apple or cranberry juice

Bread sticks

Low-fat yogurt with fresh fruit

Dehydrated soup made with water plus nonfat dry milk

Mix of raisins, dried pineapple cubes, toasted whole-grain bread cubes

Celery sticks with low-fat ricotta cheese

Low-fat cottage cheese whipped in blender with dried onions, vegetable flakes, herbs, and Worcestershire or soy sauce— use as a dip or spread on whole-grain crackers

Ice milk

Small cans of tuna fish packed in water

Graham crackers

Bowl of vegetable chunks; pepper, cherry tomatoes, cucumber, zucchini, green beans

Bowl of fresh fruit chunks (serve with toothpicks: apple, pear, fresh pineapple, peaches, melon, strawberries, grapes)

Note: Nuts and seeds are very high in fat. Leave them out of your snacks unless you make up for them by cutting down on your fat in other areas of your diet!

Smokers

Though smoking is a far greater factor in your cancer risk than is diet, eating habits can help you to protect yourself somewhat from the effects of smoking on your cancer risk.

For reasons that nobody pretends to understand, dietary cholesterol appears to interact with smoking to raise the risk of lung cancer significantly, especially for men.

Thus, if you're a man who just can't quit smoking, you should make a determined effort to bring down your dietary cholesterol as much as possible.

And since eating fruits and vegetables high in beta-carotene and vitamin C has been found to reduce lung cancer risk in smokers, no matter how many cigarettes they smoke each day, it may be that smokers will benefit more than nonsmokers from the anticancer life-style. Don't forget that vitamin A is crucial in the normal growth and development of the epithelial tissue that lines the lung. That's the tissue that gives rise to lung cancer.

A smoker could do himself a big favor by snacking on carrots and eating grapefruit every moment his mouth isn't actually busy with a cigarette.

Brown-Bag Lunchers

You can get better nutrition at lower cost when you pack home-baked breads, cookies, and pastries than when you rely on high-fat items like potato chips, doughnuts, and commercial cakes. At the same time, you'll be reinforcing good health habits and high standards for eating.

Use the *best* bread for sandwiches—homemade if you have the time, whole grain in any event. If you decide to bake your own bread, and it's not a bad way to get children interested in "dark" bread if they're used to eating the soft white kind, let the kids help in the baking. I know a teenage boy who's taken over the family baking himself, and who turns out a mighty fine loaf. Encourage your baking youngsters to experiment with adding such extras as raisins, nuts, or cooked wheat berries.

Raw carrots are a big favorite with youngsters and belong in the lunch box every day. For variety, cut them in different shapes: sticks, diagonals, "crinkles" cut with the wavy-edged blade you can get in most houseware departments. Include dark-green pepper rings or strips, cucumber spears (with skin left on), and zucchini slices now and then.

Some children just don't like raw carrots. If yours don't, add carrot shreds to coleslaw and tuna- and chicken-salad sandwich spreads, bake shredded or mashed carrots into brownies and cookies, even those you make from a mix.

As an alternative to sandwiches, send hot foods to school in a wide-mouth insulated container. Leftovers, thick soups, and pasta dishes lend themselves nicely to brown-bagging. Pack cold foods in those little plastic tubs that margarine comes in. Salads, marinated leftover vegetables, cottage cheese mixed with fresh fruits, raisins, nuts, and flavored with a little clove or cinnamon.

Middle Eastern pita bread is fun as a container for sandwich fillings. It's flat, circular, and opens up like an English muffin to form a little pouch to hold other foods. Try to get the whole-wheat kind, and fill it with meat bits, fish flakes, chopped vegetables, but *don't* add dressing or moist ingredients if many hours must elapse between preparing the lunch and eating it. Instead, pack the sauce, salad, oil, or other runny ingredients separately in a little plastic container and add it at lunchtime.

When making tuna, chicken, ham, or egg salad, avoid using mayonnaise or high-fat dressing. If you don't like the low-fat dressings, you can moisten foods with yogurt, low-fat cottage cheese, or even a few drops of skim milk. Work in as many vegetables as you can (celery, cucumber, shredded carrots, green pepper, cooked beets, diced zucchini, or summer squash). These add fiber and vitamins, and enable you to make a filling meal with limited-protein food. Some older children and adults prefer to pack these salads in margarine tubs, for spreading on Scandinavian whole-grain flatbread or other crackers, instead of as the filling in traditional sandwiches. (Be sure to pack a plastic knife if you choose this style of lunch!)

For variety in sandwich fillings, try:

- Low-fat cottage cheese and pineapple
- Peanut butter, banana, and sunflower seeds
- Peanut butter, raisins, and sliced apples
- Skim-milk cheese, tomato, and green pepper
- Neufchatel cheese, pimientos, scallions, and anchovies

Alternatives to sandwiches:

- Chicken wings (see recipe)
- Hunan spicy beef (see recipe)
- Greek meatballs (see recipe)
- Tomatoes or raw green peppers stuffed with tuna or cottage cheese
- Low-fat quiche, made with ricotta cheese and egg whites baked in small aluminum pans (you don't have to line them with pastry)

Dieters
The eating patterns suggested in this book are intended for people who want to *maintain* their present weight, and aren't

meant to help you gain or lose. Diets designed to bring your weight into the proper range are different from those structured to keep you where you are, and involve stresses and metabolic changes that need to be monitored.

If you're not satisfied with your weight, go to a physician and get professional help. If your family doctor isn't interested in counseling you on a continuing basis, taking blood and urine samples to make sure your body is functioning properly, ask to be referred to an internist with a special interest in diet and nutrition.

Dieters have special problems. A physician who's treated many of them knows how to handle the psychology, as well as the physiology, of gaining or losing. He or she knows how to keep you motivated, and can spot early signs of trouble. Don't attempt to gain or lose more than a few pounds on your own. Your body is a delicate mechanism, and abrupt, significant changes in what you consume can cause you harm.

Diets which involve very high protein or very low calories in particular need a doctor's supervision. These are deliberately unbalanced, in order to achieve the short-term goal of restoring your weight to normal. They're not meant as a way of life. You can take risks—like the low fiber and high fat of a high-protein diet—for a little while. But don't do it on your own.

When you reach your desired weight, the Everyday Food Plans can help you maintain it, while giving you all the other benefits of balanced, varied, moderate nutrition.

19
Some Sample Menus and Recipes

1,600 Calories

Breakfast
>   6 ounces orange juice
>   1 slice whole-grain bread
>   2 teaspoons margarine or butter
>   ½ cup oatmeal with 2 teaspoons sugar
>   1 cup low-fat milk

Lunch
>   chicken sandwich: 2 slices whole-wheat bread, lettuce, tomato slices, 2 ounces chicken, 2 teaspoons mayonnaise
>   ½ cup coleslaw (cabbage and carrot shreds)
>   1 cup low-fat milk

Dinner
>   3 ounces lean, trimmed roast beef
>   1 medium baked potato with 2 teaspoons sour cream
>   1 cup spinach salad with low-fat dressing
>   1 small biscuit (made with white enriched flour) with 1 teaspoon butter

Snack
>   2 graham crackers

2,000 Calories

Breakfast

½ grapefruit
1 soft-boiled egg
2 slices whole-grain toast
2 teaspoons margarine or butter and
    1 teaspoon jelly or jam
1 cup low-fat milk

Lunch

1 cup split-pea soup
stuffed tomato: 1 medium tomato, 2 ounces water-
    packed tuna, chopped celery, onion, green pepper,
    2 teaspoons dressing
6 small rye crackers
½ cup frozen yogurt (counts as 4 teaspoons sugar plus
    1 cup low-fat milk)

Dinner

3 ounces lean, trimmed pork chop
1 cup broccoli
1 cup rice with 1 teaspoon parsley butter
½ cup chopped apples with 2 teaspoons curried
    mayonnaise, on bed of lettuce
1 glass white wine (count as 6 teaspoons sugar)

Snack

1½ ounces natural cheese
4 whole-grain crackers
1 pear

2,400 Calories

Breakfast

½ cup stewed apricots
2 whole-grain pancakes with 3 teaspoons butter and
    2 teaspoons syrup
1 cup low-fat milk

Lunch

> 3 ounces hamburger, 1 slice American cheese, lettuce,
> sliced tomato, on hamburger roll
> 6 carrot sticks
> 1 peach

Dinner

> 4 ounces broiled bluefish
> 1 medium potato, boiled, with 2 teaspoons butter and
> sprinkling of fresh dill
> 1 cup boiled beets
> 1 cup green salad with low-fat dressing
> 4 oatmeal cookies (count as 5 teaspoons sugar plus
> 2 slices bread)

Snack

> 1 apple
> Nut bread sandwich with 4 teaspoons cream cheese

2,800 Calories

Breakfast

> 6 ounces grapefruit juice
> 1 cup oatmeal with ¼ cup raisins, 2 teaspoons
> sugar
> 1 slice whole-grain toast, with 1 teaspoon butter or
> margarine, 1 teaspoon jam
> 1 cup whole milk

Lunch

> 2 turkey sandwiches: 4 slices white enriched bread,
> 3 ounces sliced turkey with skin removed, lettuce,
> sliced red onion, 2 teaspoons mayonnaise
> 1 cup low-fat ratatouille (see recipe)
> 1 cup whole milk
> ½ cup frozen yogurt

Dinner

4 ounces Hunan spicy beef (see recipe)
1 cup boiled rice
¾ cup steamed carrots and broccoli
1 large dinner roll with 2 teaspoons margarine
½ cup sliced fresh pineapple
12 ounces beer (count as 10 teaspoons sugar)

Snack

peanut butter sandwich: 2 teaspoons peanut butter,
2 teaspoons jelly, 2 slices whole-wheat toast
1 medium bunch grapes

A Note on the Recipes

These recipes are based on the principles inherent in the NAS guidelines on diet, nutrition, and cancer, on the tips and techniques outlined in this book, and, perhaps most important, on my own experience in the kitchen and on the likes and dislikes of my family and friends. Their purpose is twofold: to provide you with some new dishes so you can see for yourself that a balanced, varied, moderate diet is not only healthy but practical and enjoyable, *and* to stimulate your own creative thinking about the food you eat.

None of these recipes call for salt. If you find, at the end of preparing a dish, that it needs salting, add a little, but if you're not stingy with spices and seasonings, you may well find salt isn't necessary. In no case should you dash the salt onto the food automatically. Taste it!

Trim the meat in each recipe before you start cooking—preferably just after you take it from the refrigerator, when the fat is still solid and easy to see. Peel the skin from chicken, game hens, and other poultry before you cook it. The only exception is whole roast turkey, which is cooked with the skin on, to be removed from each portion as it's carved from the hot or cold bird.

Don't peel vegetables or fruits, except for the thick-skinned types like oranges or avocadoes. And, with obvious exceptions like peach pits and squash seeds, don't remove seeds.

The number of servings refers to the Everyday Food Plans, and the serving size of some of the meat dishes may seem undersized by regular standards. Please remember that the menus derived from the Food Plans include additional foods which make each meal generous and filling. If you're not following the Food Plans, you may want to increase the serving size, depending on the other foods to be served in the meal.

By consulting the Trade-Offs, you can get a good approximation of the way that dishes combining ingredients from several food groups fit into the day's total nutrition. You need not figure it out to the last calorie, but it is a good idea to keep track of the fat, sugar, milk-group, and grain-group equivalents as you use them up throughout the day.

Swedish Cabbage Soup
(4 Servings)

    1 medium cabbage
    2 tablespoons corn oil
    3 quarts stock
   10 peppercorns

Cube the cabbage, cutting away the tough parts, and cook very gently in the oil in a covered pot. (At this point, Swedes traditionally add 1 tablespoon dark-brown sugar.) When the cabbage is golden-colored, add the stock and peppercorns and simmer 2 to 3 hours, until the cabbage is extremely tender.

Variation: Make tiny, grape-sized meatballs out of ½ pound ground veal, 1 egg white, 2 tablespoons bran, 1 tablespoon Worcestershire, ¼ teaspoon nutmeg, and add to the soup during the last 10 minutes of cooking. If you double the meatball recipe, the soup becomes a meat dish; serve it with whole-grain bread, a salad, and a simple dessert like clafoutis for a nice Sunday night supper.

Ad Hoc Vegetable Soup
(10-12 Servings)

The ingredients for this soup depend on what's available, either as odds and ends in your refrigerator or as vegetables bought for the purpose from your produce department. I assume that you have the first three ingredients on hand—from there on, the composition of the soup is up to you. To my mind, a good soup is spontaneous, almost a Zen happening— specially created for the moment, and never the same twice.

> 1 cup white wine
> 1 large onion, chopped
> 3 celery stalks, with leaves, chopped
> 1 cup green fresh parsley or dill, or a combination of the two
> 2–3 carrots, chopped or grated
> 3 cups vegetables, fresh, frozen, or canned
> 1–2 medium potatoes, cut in spoon-sized pieces
> 3 quarts stock

Heat the wine in the bottom of a large pot. Add the onion and celery stalks and cook and stir until vegetables are soft. Add the other ingredients and the stock, and simmer quietly for about 2 hours.

Your vegetable choices are infinite. The obvious ones are canned beans or tomatoes, leftover cooked vegetables of all kinds, cabbage, and every variety of greens. But don't overlook other possibilities: broccoli or cauliflower stems, peeled and cubed; pumpkin and other deep-yellow squashes (cut in *small* cubes so they won't take forever to cook). Turnips. Beets. The tag ends of cucumbers. The good half of a tomato that's going soft on one side.

Of course you can add rice, pasta, and whole grains— quick-cooking oatmeal makes a lovely thickener for vegetable soups. But if your ad hoc soup is a big one, intended to last for several meals, don't add starchy ingredients like pasta or rice to the whole potful. Instead, take out as much soup as you'll need for the meal at hand and add the noodles, barley, or whatever to just the amount you intend to serve right away. This measure will keep the starch from turning soggy when the leftover soup is stored in the refrigerator, and gives you the opportunity to vary the character of the soup from meal to meal by adding different special ingredients.

"Cream" Soups
(4 Servings)

Bean curd makes these soups thick and rich textured, but adds no flavor of its own—and no fat at all. Just good vegetable protein, which, when completed with whole-grain bread, makes the centerpiece of a satisfying meatless meal.

> 1 cup cooked vegetables (broccoli, cauliflower, carrots, green beans, pumpkin, tomatoes, etc.)
> 1 onion, grated, cooked in ½ cup white wine
> 2 cakes bean curd
> 2 cups broth (chicken, beef, or vegetable, with fat skimmed off)

Blend the cooked vegetables in food processor or blender till smooth and add the onion cooked in wine. Blend again. Break the bean curd in pieces and add to container, blend till smooth. Add the broth a little at a time and blend till smooth. For a hot soup, pour in saucepan and heat gently; for a cold soup, chill in refrigerator for one hour.

Try these variations:
- Pumpkin, flavored with nutmeg and grated fresh ginger
- Green beans with basil
- Carrot with cumin or curry powder
- Broccoli with garlic (cook along with the onion in the wine), garnished with chopped pimiento

Bean Soup
(4 Servings as main dish, 8 Servings as first course)

> 1 pound Yankee beans, lima beans, chick-peas, or other dried beans
> ¼ cup olive oil
> 1 large onion, chopped
> 2 cloves garlic, minced
> pepper
> 1 6-ounce can tomato purée or 1-pound can tomatoes
> 3 quarts water
> 1 teaspoon dried herb (mint, oregano, thyme, or savory)

Soak the beans overnight in water to cover. Add oil, onion, garlic, pepper, and tomato purée or tomatoes to the 3 quarts water and the beans. Simmer for about 2 hours or until the beans are tender. Add the herb in the last 15 minutes of cooking.

Beef or Lamb with Cabbage
(4 Servings)

   1¼ pounds lean beef or lamb, with all fat trimmed
    1 tablespoon butter
    1 tablespoon corn oil
    3 onions, chopped
    1 cup tomato sauce
    1 cup water
    1 large head of savoy cabbage
      pepper
      lemon slices

Cut the meat into 2-inch cubes, and brown well in the oil and butter. Add onions, cook 5 minutes over low heat. Add tomato sauce, water, cabbage, pepper, bring to a boil. Cover and simmer 1 hour, or until meat is tender; add lemon slices during last 15 minutes.

Chicken and Sauerkraut
(4 Servings)

    1 chicken (fryer or broiler), cut in serving pieces
    2 tablespoons corn oil
    1 tablespoon butter
      pepper
    2 onions, chopped
    1 cup celery, chopped
    1 one-pound can tomatoes
    1 pound sauerkraut
   ½ lemon, sliced
    2 sticks cinnamon

Brown the chicken lightly in the oil and butter, using a deep pot. Grind a little pepper over the pieces, and add onions and celery. Cook 5 minutes over low heat, add tomatoes. Rinse the sauerkraut with cold water, add to the pot with lemon slices and cinnamon sticks. Simmer very gently for 1 to 1½ hours.

Greek Fish with Walnut Sauce
(4 Servings)

    ½ cup olive oil
    1 tablespoon unbleached flour
    1 teaspoon paprika
    1 quart warm water
    1 3-pound sea bass
    1 cup walnuts
    1 clove garlic, chopped
    ¼ cup chopped parsley

Heat oil, sprinkle in the flour, cook and stir till brown. Add paprika and slowly stir in the water. Add the fish and simmer 10 minutes for each inch of thickness. (A fish 2 inches thick should cook for 20 minutes.) Allow fish to cool in the liquid.

In blender or food processor, grind the walnuts and garlic. Add a teaspoon or two of the fish broth to make a smooth paste, and gradually work in a cup of broth. Transfer the fish to a hot platter and pour the walnut sauce over. Sprinkle with chopped parsley.

Lamb in Packages
(4 Servings)

An alternative to grilled hamburgers for the backyard barbecue.

> 1¼ pounds lamb (any cut), cut in 5-ounce serving pieces
> garlic to taste, cut in slivers
> ½ pound mild feta cheese
> 2 carrots, cut in thin strips
> 4 small onions, peeled
> 2 stalks celery, each cut in 4 pieces
> 2 medium potatoes, cooked and halved
> 4 slices lemon
> 1 teaspoon dried mint or oregano
> lemon juice

For each serving, use a square of aluminum foil. On each place a piece of lamb, pierced with the tip of a knife and garlic slivers inserted. To each piece of lamb, add a 2-ounce cube of cheese, ¼ of the carrot sticks, an onion, 2 pieces of celery, half a potato, a slice of lemon, a pinch of mint or oregano, and a squeeze of lemon juice. Fold the foil around the meat and vegetables and seal with a double fold like a package. Put the packages on a baking sheet and cook 2 hours in a 350° oven, or on a backyard grill with a baking pan inverted over them to keep the heat in. Let each person open his own package on his plate.

Stir-Fry Meat with Vegetables
(4 Servings)

> 1 pound lean boneless meat (flank steak, round steak; fresh pork; lamb shoulder; veal; chicken or turkey breast), cubed or sliced thinly against the grain

Marinade:

- 2 tablespoons cold water
- 2 tablespoons soy sauce
- 2 teaspoons cornstarch
- 4 tablespoons peanut oil
- 5–6 cups fresh vegetables (broccoli, cauliflower, green beans, scallions, green peppers, snow pea pods, green or sweet red peppers, spinach leaves, mustard greens, etc.; carrots must be parboiled)
- ½ teaspoon sugar
- 2 tablespoons rice wine or dry sherry
- 1 teaspoon cornstarch plus 2 tablespoons water

Trim all fat from meat, remove skin from poultry.

Mix meat with the marinade.

Heat a skillet or a wok and add 2 tablespoons oil, add the vegetables and stir-fry 5 minutes, remove and set aside. Wipe the pan with paper towel and reheat, add the rest of the oil. Add the meat-marinade mixture, stir-fry, stirring carefully to separate the pieces, and add the sugar, sherry or rice wine. Add the cooked vegetables, stirring while they heat through. Thicken with the cornstarch-and-water mixture, stirring the meat and vegetables until the sauce becomes clear.

Greek Meatballs
(4 Servings)

A nice meaty prelude to a meal with a main dish that's meatless. These meatballs are good served hot, and excellent cold. Try them as a brown-bag lunch, in a plastic container.

1 pound chopped beef
½ cup whole-wheat bread crumbs
2 egg whites
1 teaspoon Dijon mustard
¼ cup chopped parsley
1 medium onion, grated
1 clove garlic, chopped fine
1 teaspoon dried mint
¼ teaspoon dried oregano
1 teaspoon Worcestershire sauce
pinch each of allspice, cinnamon, and cloves
½ cup tomato sauce
¼ cup water
1 teaspoon grated lemon rind

Mix all the ingredients except the last three. Shape into one-inch balls and put on nonstick baking pan. Bake in 450° oven for 20 minutes and drain on paper towels.

In a saucepan, simmer tomato sauce, water, and lemon peel for 5 minutes. Add meatballs to sauce and store in covered container in refrigerator overnight. Serve hot or cold.

Stuffed Whole Cabbage
(4 Servings)

A spectacular way to serve the king of the cruciferae. You need a *big* pot.

1 large savoy (green) cabbage
2 pounds of Swiss chard, parboiled, drained, and chopped
1 pound lean fresh pork, ground
2 medium onions, chopped fine
1 tablespoon corn oil
1 clove garlic, peeled and chopped fine
1 cup canned tomatoes, drained and chopped
½ cup brown rice, cooked and drained
½ teaspoon nutmeg
1 teaspoon savory
enough beef or chicken stock to cover

Take off the outer leaves of the cabbage, slice off the bottom of the stem and parboil it in a large pot for 10 to 15 minutes. Drain and cool.

Put the cabbage in the center of a square of cheesecloth about 18″ on each side (a clean piece of an old sheet will do) and gently spread about 18 or 20 of the outer leaves, leaving them attached to the cabbage at their base. You will end up with something that looks like a big green rose in bloom.

Remove the tightly wrapped heart of the cabbage by slicing horizontally across the core, leaving the base that the outer leaves are attached to.

Chop the leaves of the heart of the cabbage, discarding the tough core. Squeeze them to remove moisture, and mix with all the other ingredients. Mold the mixture into a compact ball, put it in the center of the opened-out cabbage, and, one by one, put the leaves of the cabbage back around it.

Now bring the corners of the cloth square together so the cabbage is neatly enclosed, tie it up with a piece of string, and place it in the bottom of your pot. Cover it with stock (plain water plus bouillon cubes will do) and cook, loosely covered, simmering very gently, about 3 to 4 hours.

I bring this splendid dish to the table still wrapped in its cloth, resting in a big earthenware salad bowl, since the ceremony of unwrapping it adds to everybody's pleasure. The simplest way to serve it is to cut the cabbage into quarters with a stout knife, from the crown through the core, lifting each quarter out with two big spoons.

Variation: For the tomatoes and seasonings, substitute ½ cup chopped scallions, ½ cup chopped water chestnuts, 2 tablespoons light soy sauce, 1 tablespoon fresh ginger.

West Coast Salad
(4 Servings)

This dish from western Sweden is as fancy or as frugal as you want to make it.

2 cups cooked seafood (crabmeat, scallops cut in small pieces, diced shrimp, lobster for luxury; flaked cooked flounder, sea bass, tile for everyday; canned tuna or salmon for convenience. A combination of several types of fish is tastiest. For real economy, use half seafood and half diced bean curd).
1 cup cooked corn
1 cucumber, seeded and diced
1 tomato, seeded and diced
1 cup diced celery
1 cup diced carrots
½ cup chopped scallions
½ cup chopped fresh dill
2 tablespoons lemon juice
½ head of iceberg lettuce, torn in bits

Mix all ingredients except lettuce. Put lettuce in bottom of bowl and heap the vegetable-seafood mixture on top.

Salade de Boeuf
(4 Servings)

1 pound lean beef, trimmed of visible fat and boiled with onion, celery, bay leaf
8 very small boiled potatoes, in skins
1 pound green beans, cooked
2 tomatoes, cut in wedges
1 red onion, sliced
1 head romaine lettuce
2 scallions, chopped (optional)

Cut the beef in small cubes; cut each potato in half, and arrange with other ingredients on a bed of romaine, torn in small pieces.

Serve with:
Red Wine Dressing
½ cup red wine
1 tablespoon Dijon-type prepared mustard
ground black pepper
½ teaspoon thyme
½ teaspoon basil
¼ cup fresh parsley, chopped fine

Put all ingredients in a covered jar and shake briskly until well blended.

Beef Tacos
(6 Servings, 2 tacos each)

1 cup chopped tomato
1 cup shredded lettuce
½ cup (2 oz.) natural cheddar cheese
1 pound ground lean beef
½ cup chopped onion
8 ounce can tomato sauce
2 teaspoons chili powder
12 cooked taco shells

Mix tomato, lettuce, and cheese and set aside.

Brown the beef and onion in a nonstick frying pan and drain the excess fat. Stir in the tomato sauce and chili powder. Bring to a boil. Reduce heat and cook 10 to 15 minutes, uncovered, stirring occasionally. When mixture is dry and crumbly, divide it among the taco shells, and add about two tablespoons of the tomato-lettuce-cheese mixture to each.

Chicken Wings
(4 Servings)

The inexpensive wing is the most flavorful part of the chicken. Cut off the tips and discard, and separate the other two bones at the joint.

Basic Recipe
4 pounds chicken wings
2 quarts water

Bring the water to a boil and add the chicken wings, cut in pieces. Cook for 3 minutes or until the skin becomes firm and yellow. Drain, cool, and slip the skin off each piece. Before cooking more, shake the wings with one of the three coating combinations below. Then put the wings on a wire rack in a shallow pan in the oven and cook 10 minutes at 450°.

Buffalo Style: Put 2 tablespoons Tabasco sauce and ½

teaspoon sugar in large jar or plastic container, add the chicken wings and shake well. Cook.

After cooking, serve with a blender dip made from 1 oz. blue cheese, 2 bean curd cakes, ½ medium onion, grated, thinned with a little chicken broth, and with plenty of celery and carrot sticks.

Garlic and Herb: Shake the chicken wings with a combination of ½ cup white wine, 2 cloves garlic, crushed, ½ teaspoon peanut oil, black pepper, ½ teaspoon basil, ½ teaspoon oregano, ½ teaspoon thyme. Cook. Serve with French or Italian bread, raw green pepper spears.

Chinese Style: Shake the chicken wings with 2 tablespoons soy sauce, 2 cloves garlic, crushed, 2 teaspoons grated fresh ginger, 1 tablespoon dry sherry. Cook. Serve with fresh broccoli spears and scallions.

Chicken or Turkey Pâté
(Makes one loaf, about 2 pounds)

- ½ cup plus 1 tablespoon nonfat dry milk
- 1 teaspoon white pepper
- ½ teaspoon ground ginger
- ½ teaspoon ground nutmeg
- 2 shallots or 1 small onion
- 1 pound chicken breast or turkey thigh meat, skinned and boned
- 1¼ cups chicken broth, frozen to a mush

Mix ½ cup dry milk with spices. In a food processor, chop the onion and poultry meat, add the spice mixture, and the frozen chicken broth, gradually. Empty the mixture into a loaf pan (either nonstick or sprayed with lubricant), packing the mixture firmly with a rubber spatula to avoid pockets of air, and bake in a very slow oven (250°) for 1 hour and 45 minutes. After the first hour, brush the top with a glaze made from 2 tablespoons water and the remaining nonfat dry milk. Cool the pâté after removing from oven, then chill in refrigerator at least 2 hours. The texture improves if you chill it for a day or two.

You can substitute very lean, trimmed beef for the chicken

or turkey, using 1 cup beef broth plus ½ cup brandy instead of the chicken broth.

Fish (haddock, flounder, canned salmon with bones and skin removed) can also substitute for the poultry, using 1 cup chicken broth plus ½ cup white wine. Fish pâtés are even better when you add ½ cup fresh dill, very finely chopped— but if you can't find the fresh herb, don't bother using the dried form.

Hunan Spicy Beef
(4 Servings)

This peppery dish has no gravy, since the moisture and spices cook into the thin strips of beef. It's therefore ideal as a finger food, to serve with your before-dinner drink or to pack in a plastic container for a brown-bag lunch. It will keep for about two weeks in a covered jar in the refrigerator.

This recipe makes 4 main-dish servings, 8 if used as finger food before a meal with another high-protein dish.

  ½ cup corn or peanut oil
  2 teaspoons red chili pepper, crushed
 4–6 slices fresh ginger
  ¼ teaspoon black peppercorns (or Szechwan pepper, if you can get it)
  2 cloves garlic, minced
  2 pounds lean beef (flank steak, round steak, etc.) cut in thin slices
  2 tablespoons rice wine or dry sherry
  ½ cup soy sauce

Pour the oil in a hot saucepan or wok, add the chili and ginger slices, fry until the chili darkens, and add the peppercorns, garlic, and beef. Cook over medium-high heat till the beef loses its red color, add the wine and soy sauce, and cover. Cook about 20 minutes, stirring occasionally, until the sauce has cooked away. I like to sprinkle this dish with chopped scallions or fresh coriander to add some color. It's good either hot or cold.

Hot Granola
(4 Servings)

   1 cup whole-wheat berries
   1 cup brown rice
   1 cup barley
   3 cups water or stock
   1 tablespoon oil
   1 small onion, chopped
   1 cup mushrooms, sliced
     pepper, herbs to taste

Heat the water or stock to boiling and add the whole-wheat berries. Cook at high heat for ½ hour. Reduce heat and add brown rice and barley, and continue to cook until grains are cooked but not mushy. Cover and continue cooking at moderate heat. Cook the onion in the oil until soft, add the mushrooms, and cook gently 5 to 10 minutes. Add to the cooked grains, along with the seasonings. (Savory is nice if this dish is to be served with beef; rosemary harmonizes with lamb or veal. Add allspice and a small chopped apple if this is to accompany pork.) The total cooking time may vary, depending on the individual batches of grains (this may have to do with the storage conditions). I find that 1¼ hours from start to finish is about average. You can vary the combinations of grain. Wild rice can be substituted for all or part of the brown—even a few grains add a special touch.

French Dressing
(4 Servings, with mixed green salad)

The *véritable* vinaigrette, updated.

   1½ tablespoons olive oil
   1½ tablespoons corn oil
   1 scant tablespoon red wine vinegar
   1 teaspoon Dijon-type mustard
   3–4 twists of the peppermill

Mix thoroughly with a fork, pour over salad greens.

Variations: If you want a garlicky fragrance, rub the salad bowl well with a peeled clove of garlic—adding chopped garlic or squeezing from a garlic press overpowers what should be a subtle, simple dressing.

Mash 8 to 10 green peppercorns in the mixing bowl before you add other ingredients.

For extra-low-fat vinaigrette, use 1½ tablespoons water instead of the corn oil. The olive oil is what provides the flavor, anyway.

Spinach and Brown Rice
(4 Servings)

It sounds Spartan, but it's delicious and very satisfying. Try it!

    2 tablespoons olive oil
    2 large onions, chopped
    1 teaspoon tomato paste
    2 packages frozen chopped spinach
    1 cup water
      pepper
    1 teaspoon dried herb (mint, oregano, thyme)
    1 cup brown rice, cooked 15 minutes in water

Heat the oil in a heavy pan, cook onions till golden. Add tomato paste, spinach, and water to cover. Bring to a boil, add seasonings, stir in the half-cooked rice quickly, cover, and simmer until rice is completely cooked.

Chick-Peas and Swiss Chard
(4 Servings)

Something wonderful to do with the green part of the chard. Save the white ribs for the French recipe on page 222.

        2 pounds Swiss chard
          water
        1 large (1 lb.) can chick-peas (garbanzos) or 10
          ounces dried chick-peas, cooked according to pack-
          age instructions
        1 large carrot, peeled, grated
        ⅓ cup olive oil
        1 cup canned tomatoes, drained and chopped
        4 cloves garlic, cut in slivers
        ½ cup chopped fresh dill or parsley
       12 blanched almonds
        2 eggs, hard-boiled
          dash of Tabasco
        2 tablespoons lemon juice
          whole-wheat bread crumbs

If you use dried chick-peas, soak overnight and follow
package instructions. Cook the chard lightly in boiling water
for 3 minutes, drain. Cook the tomatoes and grated carrot in
enough olive oil to cover the bottom of the pan, with the
garlic and dill or parsley for 15 minutes over low heat. In a
blender or food processor, work the almonds and the yolk of one
egg into a paste with the Tabasco and lemon juice, and add a
few chick-peas and some of their cooking liquid or juice from
the can, to create a sauce. Add the chick-peas, the almond-egg
mixture, the cooked chard, and the egg whites, sliced, to the
tomato mixture, and pour into an ovenproof dish. Sprinkle the
surface with the bread crumbs and pour the rest of the olive oil
over the surface before baking ½ hour in a hot (450°) oven.

Cauliflower Loaf
(4 Servings as a main dish, 6 Servings as an appetizer or side
dish)

        2 small cauliflowers or one large one, broken into
          florets
        4 egg whites
        ⅔ cup low-fat milk
        ½ cup grated cheese (low-fat American is fine;
          add a tablespoon grated Parmesan if you like)
        1 teaspoon Tabasco
        1 tablespoon corn oil

Steam or parboil the cauliflower and drain it well, then purée it in a food processor or put it through a hand-cranked vegetable mill. Mix the purée with the other ingredients, pour into a nonstick baking dish, and bake 20 minutes at 450°.

If you like, you can sprinkle some of the cheese on top before baking.

Red Cabbage
(4 Servings)

Soak 4 cups of chopped red cabbage in cold water for ½ hour and drain. Chop 2 or 3 onions and cook lightly in ½ cup white wine or gin. Add 3 large unpeeled apples, chopped, and cook 5 minutes over low heat. Add the chopped cabbage and 1 cup of water or apple cider. Cook for about an hour, stirring often. Add ⅓ cup vinegar and cook another 10 minutes before serving.

Baked Eggplant
(4 Servings)

The simplest and one of the best ways I know to cook this delicious—but not very nutritious—vegetable.

    2 medium eggplants
    4 cloves garlic, cut lengthwise into thin slices
    2 tablespoons olive oil
       freshly ground black pepper

Cut the eggplants lengthwise. With a sharp, long-bladed knife, cut 6 to 8 gashes in the cut surface of the eggplant, and push a slice of garlic into each. Pour the olive oil into a shallow dish—a platter is ideal—and put the eggplant halves, cut side down, in the oil. When the oil is absorbed, put the eggplant cut side up in a pan in the oven, sprinkle with pepper, and bake at 450° for 30 to 40 minutes, till the eggplant is soft and brown on top.

Carrot Pudding
(4 Servings)

2 pounds carrots, grated in a food processor or by
   hand
1 tablespoon butter
1 tablespoon corn oil
2 tablespoons lemon juice
1 teaspoon sugar (optional)
  water
1½ cups whole milk
1 egg plus 4 egg whites
  pepper, nutmeg, allspice to taste

Put the carrots, butter, oil, lemon juice, sugar (if used),
and just enough water to cover the carrots in a saucepan,
bring to a boil, and simmer, covered, for about 25 minutes.
Uncover, raise the heat, and cook rapidly to evaporate the
liquid, stirring constantly with a wooden spoon. Cool.

Combine the other ingredients with an egg beater, mix with
the cooled carrots, and bake in an ovenproof dish sprayed
with nonstick lubricant for about 30 minutes, or until the
pudding has puffed up and browned. A sprinkle of Parmesan
cheese before putting it in the oven is a nice touch.

Variations: You can cook many vegetables in main-dish
puddings like this one. Try chopped broccoli, cauliflower,
cabbage, or zucchini. For most, a simple steaming for 5 to 10
minutes is enough preparation before adding to the egg mixture.

Braised Green Beans
(4 Servings)

1 pound fresh green beans
1 tablespoon olive oil
1 tablespoon corn oil
1 clove garlic, chopped
1 large onion, quartered and sliced
2 tablespoons tomato paste
2 fresh tomatoes, peeled, seeded, and chopped coarsely
½ cup fresh parsley
  dash of Tabasco

Wash the beans and cut off the stems and ends, cut large beans in half. Heat the oil in a heavy pan, cook garlic and onion gently till golden. Add tomato paste and fresh tomatoes, simmer till slightly thickened. Add the beans, parsley, and Tabasco, cover and cook till beans are tender, about 15 minutes if fresh or 10 minutes if frozen.

Serve hot as a side dish, or cold as an appetizer or salad. When I serve them cold, I like to add 3 or 4 chopped anchovies and a tablespoon of white vinegar.

Fat-Free Ratatouille
(8 Servings)

This classic Provençal French dish is usually made with lots of olive oil, but this oil-free version is equally good. If you miss the flavor of the oil, put a few drops of the strongly flavored Greek olive oil on each serving at the table.

½ cup white wine
2 cloves garlic, crushed
2 onions, chopped
1 medium eggplant, cubed
1 cup tomatoes (fresh, seeded, and chopped if possible, otherwise canned tomatoes, well drained)
1 medium green pepper, cut in one-inch pieces
2 large zucchini, sliced
½ cup fresh parsley
½ cup fresh basil leaves *or* ½ teaspoon dried basil

Heat the white wine and add garlic and onions, cook uncovered, stirring constantly, until half the wine is evaporated and the onions are transparent. Add the eggplant and cook, covered, until it begins to soften. Add tomatoes and cook till eggplant is fork-tender. Drain the excess liquid into a small saucepan and boil rapidly till reduced to ½ cup. Add it with other ingredients to the eggplant-tomato mixture and cook until the zucchini slices are tender.

A favorite side dish, hot or cold, and a lovely low-calorie summer lunch, served on dark-green lettuce. You can vary it by adding:

- 1 cup cooked carrots, sliced
- ½ cup olives, sliced
- 1 cup yellow summer squash, in cubes

Chard Ribs
(4 Servings approximately)

Americans are used to eating only the green leafy parts of Swiss chard, but the French prefer the white ribs. Both parts contain the indoles and flavones we need; the greens contain vitamin C.

Boil together:

> 2 quarts water
> 1 large onion, sliced
> 2 bay leaves
> 1 tablespoon thyme
> 1 tablespoon white vinegar
> 2 anchovy fillets
> 2 large cloves garlic parsley
> Tabasco sauce
> pinch of saffron (optional)

After ½ hour, add the ribs of 2 pounds of Swiss chard, trimmed nicely, with any tough strings removed, and cut into pieces about 1 by 4 inches. Cook the ribs about 10 minutes, then remove them to an ovenproof dish. Save 2 cups of bouillon in which they cooked. Meanwhile, mash 2 anchovy fillets and two large, peeled garlic cloves. Heat 1 tablespoon olive oil with 1 tablespoon flour in a medium-sized frying pan, add the anchovy-garlic paste, a handful of chopped parsley, a few drops of Tabasco, and a pinch of saffron. Stir together and slowly add 2 cups of the liquid in which you cooked the chard ribs. Let the sauce simmer about 20 minutes. Skim it as needed. Grind some pepper over the cooked chard ribs and pour the sauce over them. Cook in a hot oven (450°) for about 20 minutes longer.

Kristin's Experimental Oatmeal Bread
(1 large loaf, or 2 small)

This is the best bread I know of.

- 1 envelope dried yeast, dissolved in 1 cup of warm water
- ½ cup low-fat milk
- 3 tablespoons butter
- 1 tablespoon honey
- ½ cup molasses
- 1 cup old-fashioned Quaker Oats
- 2 cups unbleached flour

Warm the milk over low heat, add butter, honey, and molasses and stir till butter is melted. Cool and add to yeast. Work in the oatmeal, cover with a damp cloth and allow to rise in a warm place. When doubled in bulk, punch down and add the unbleached flour. Knead on a floured board for 10 minutes, then shape into one large loaf pan or two small ones, and allow to rise again. When the dough has nearly reached the top of the pan, bake in slow oven (300°) about an hour. You can brush the top of each loaf with oil or melted butter if you like.

Whole-Grain Bread
(2 loaves)

- 2 cups unbleached white flour
- 1 envelope dry yeast
- ½ cup honey or molasses
- ¼ cup warm water
- 2 cups low-fat milk
- 3 cups whole-wheat flour
- 1 cup old-fashioned oatmeal
- 2 tablespoons butter (or polyunsaturated oil)

Sift the unbleached flour. Mix the yeast with honey or molasses and warm water, cover with a plate and let stand until foamy. Heat the milk until a skin forms on top, cool to lukewarm, stir in yeast, the whole-wheat flour and oatmeal. If you are using butter, melt it and add; or pour the oil in. Mix thoroughly and add enough of the unbleached flour to make a dough. Let stand for 10 minutes, then knead for 10 minutes on a floured board. Work in, ½ cup at a time, the unbleached flour until the dough is firm, elastic, and no longer sticky.

Shape the dough into a ball, cover the surface with a film of melted butter or oil (you need only a little bit), and place it in a large, greased bowl. Cover the dough with a damp cloth and let it stand in a warm spot until it has doubled in bulk. Divide the dough in two parts and shape each into a loaf. Put each loaf in a bread pan and brush the top with melted butter or oil. Cover with damp cloth and let the loaves rise again till they've nearly doubled in bulk. Bake at 400° for 10 minutes, then reduce heat to 375° and bake 40 minutes longer. The loaves are done when they sound hollow when you thump them with your finger.

Basic Sponge Cake

Virtually fat-free, this easy-to-make cake beats those made from a mix for its low sodium content, too.

>   1 cup white sugar, sifted
>   6 eggs
>   ¼ cup boiling water
>   1 tablespoon lemon juice
>   1 cup cake flour (this time, don't use the unbleached kind; it's just too heavy)
>   1½ teaspoons baking powder

Separate 5 eggs and discard the yolks. Beat one whole egg plus two whites until light, then add the sifted sugar and the boiling water. Cool, then beat in the lemon juice, plus additional flavorings (see below).

Sift the flour before measuring and resift with the baking powder and add gradually to the egg mixture.

Whip the remaining egg whites until stiff but not dry, and fold them into the batter. Bake the cake in an ungreased

9-inch tube pan in a 325° oven for 45-50 minutes. Invert to cool in the pan.

Variations:

Lemon or orange sponge cake: Mix 1-2 teaspoons lemon or orange rind with the sugar before adding to the egg-water mixture, and add a teaspoon lemon or orange extract along with the lemon juice.

Vanilla: Add 1½ teaspoons vanilla along with the lemon juice.

Almond: Add 1½ teaspoons almond extract with the lemon juice and sprinkle slivered almonds on the cake after it's cool.

There are lots of good alternatives to buttery frostings. Try dribbling frozen orange juice concentrate, diluted with an equal amount of water, over the cooled cake, or soak it in a simple rum syrup made by boiling ¼ cup sugar, ¼ cup rum, ¼ cup water together for 5 minutes. A simple dusting of confectioners' sugar makes the cake look elegant without adding any calories to speak of. You can fill the center of the cake with fresh fruit and arrange more fruit around the edge— it's surprising how fancy this simple dessert can be!

Brownies

The grated carrots add beta-carotene and just a suggestion of texture, something like coconut, but without the saturated fat.

>   4 oz. chocolate
>   ½ cup butter or margarine
>   1 whole egg plus 6 egg whites
>   2 cups sugar
>   1 teaspoon vanilla
>   1 cup unbleached flour
>   1 cup grated carrots
>   1 cup nut meats (use less for lower fat)

Melt the chocolate and butter together. Beat the eggs and add the sugar gradually, and fold in the chocolate-butter mixture. Add vanilla. Sift the flour into the batter and beat till smooth. Add the carrots and nut meats. Pour into a greased 9 × 13 pan, and bake at 325° for about 30 minutes. Cool in the pan and cut into squares.

Oatmeal Cookies
(Makes 12 large, 18 small cookies)

    1 cup unbleached flour
    ¼ teaspoon soda
    ½ teaspoon cinnamon
    ¼ teaspoon cloves
    ½ teaspoon nutmeg
    ⅔ cup brown sugar
    ½ cup soft margarine or butter
    2 egg whites
    ¾ cup old-fashioned rolled oats
    2 tablespoons yogurt, molasses, or buttermilk
    ¼ cup chopped nuts
    ½ cup shredded carrots
    ½ cup chopped raisins, figs, or dates

Sift the dry ingredients, and with your hands work in the brown sugar and margarine. Add the egg whites, oats, yogurt, nuts, carrots, and raisins in order. Drop the batter from a spoon onto greased and floured cookie sheets, and, with the bottom of a glass dipped in cold water, flatten each cookie. Chill. Bake at 375° for 15 to 20 minutes.

Whole-Wheat Pie Crust
(1 10-inch pie crust)

    1½ cups whole-wheat flour
    ½ teaspoon baking powder
    ½ cup less 1 tablespoon shortening (I use about ⅓
        butter, ⅓ corn-oil margarine, ⅓ hydrogenated
        vegetable shortening)
    ⅓ cup cold water (not ice water)

Sift the flour, measure, and add baking powder. Sift again into mixing bowl, and turn the "siftings" remaining in the sieve into the bowl. (Sifting is for measuring accuracy and to lighten the texture of the flour, not to remove the good fiber in the whole-wheat flour!)

Blend in the shortening with 2 forks or a pastry cutter.

226

Pinch a bit of the mixture between your fingers; if it doesn't hold together, add a little more margarine.

Sprinkle the cold water on the flour mixture and mix lightly with your fingers. Dust the pastry board with just enough flour to cover the surface. Roll out the dough as thinly as possible, and use as you would ordinary pie crust.

Note: Whole-wheat pie crust behaves differently from white-flour crust during the rolling and handling, and will probably seem unusually stiff. I suggest you try it once or twice for informal family meals before making a whole-wheat crust for a company dinner. It's not difficult, but some people find it takes some getting used to.

Pumpkin or Squash Pie
(1 10-inch pie)

1 recipe whole-wheat pie crust
1 package frozen pumpkin or squash
4 egg whites
1 cup skim milk
½ cup dark-brown sugar
¼ teaspoon ground ginger
¼ teaspoon cloves
¼ teaspoon nutmeg
¼ teaspoon cinnamon
¼ cup grated carrots (optional)

Line a 10-inch pie pan with whole-wheat pie crust. Combine the pumpkin and other ingredients, mix very thoroughly, and fill the crust. Bake in a moderate (350°) oven for one hour.

Clafouti
(4–6 Servings)

An extraordinarily versatile dessert, much more impressive than the simple ingredients and straightforward preparation would suggest. It's French in origin, pronounced "kla-FOO-tee."

¾ cup unbleached flour
1 whole egg plus 4 egg whites
  skim milk or water
½ pound fruit (see below)

Make a batter with the flour, eggs, and enough water or skim milk to bring it to the consistency of heavy cream. Arrange the fruit in a nonstick pan or an ordinary baking dish sprayed with lubricant, and pour the batter over. Cook for 45 minutes to 1 hour in a hot oven (400°). Serve warm or cold, with a dusting of confectioners' sugar when you want to be particularly festive.

Suggested fruits:

- Black cherries, soaked in rum, brandy, or kirsch if desired
- Sliced apples (unpeeled), sprinkled with rum or Scotch whiskey and dusted with nutmeg or cinnamon
- Sliced fresh peaches, with 1 teaspoon vanilla added to the batter, and ½ cup chopped pecans
- Sliced fresh pears, with 1 teaspoon vanilla added to batter and 1 tablespoon chocolate chips tucked among the pieces of fruit
- Orange sections arranged alternately with apple slices, with ½ cup white raisins soaked in sherry
- Bananas, sliced lengthwise, with chunks of fresh or canned pineapple

Use your imagination and whatever fresh fruits are in season. If you use berries, they should be slightly underripe; otherwise the clafouti will become too juicy and will tend to burn.

A Bouquet of Cookbooks

Many of the recipes in this book have been adapted from some appearing in these cookbooks. These books contain a wealth of exciting recipes, which, while devised before the report on diet, nutrition, and cancer was published, can be brought into conformity with the low-fat, high-fiber life-style if you apply the techniques suggested in this book.

Akerstrom, Jenny. *The Princesses' Cook Book*. New York: Albert Bonnier, 1936.

Beck, Phineas. *Clementine in the Kitchen*. New York: Hastings House, 1963.

de Groot, Roy Andries. *Feasts for All Seasons*. New York: Alfred A. Knopf, 1966.

Lin, Florence. *Florence Lin's Regional Chinese Cookbook*. New York: Hawthorne Books, 1975.

Meyers, Perla. *The Seasonal Kitchen: A Return to Fresh Foods*. New York: Holt, Rinehart and Winston, 1973.

Orton, Mildred Ellen. *Cooking with Wholegrains*. New York: Farrar, Straus & Giroux, 1973.

Olney, Richard. *Simple French Food*. New York: Atheneum, 1974.

Romagnoli, Margaret and G. Franco. *The Romagnolis' Meatless Cookbook*. Boston: Atlantic-Little, Brown, 1976.

The Women of St. Paul's Greek Orthodox Church, Hempstead, New York. *The Art of Greek Cookery*. Garden City: Doubleday, 1963.

Bibliography

Committee on Diet, Nutrition, and Cancer, Assembly of Life Sciences, Nutritional Research Council, National Academy of Sciences. *Diet, Nutrition, and Cancer*. Washington, D.C.: National Academy Press, 1982.

Committee on Diet, Nutrition, and Cancer, Assembly of Life Sciences, Nutritional Research Council, National Academy of Sciences. *Diet, Nutrition, and Cancer: Directions for Research*. Washington, D.C.: National Academy Press, 1983.

American Cancer Society, *Workshop Conference on Nutrition in Cancer Causation and Prevention*. Baltimore, Md.: Waverly Press, 1983.

American Dietetic Association. *Food 2: A Publication in Food and Nutrition*. Chicago: American Dietetic Association, 1982.

American Dietetic Association. *Food 3: A Publication in Food and Nutrition*. Chicago: American Dietetic Association, 1982.

Brody, Jane. *Jane Brody's Nutrition Book*. New York: Bantam Books, 1980.

Carper, Jean. *The Brand-Name Nutrition Counter*. New York: Bantam Books, 1980.

Curtis, Helena. *Biology*. 3rd. ed. New York: Worth Publishers, 1979.

Doll, Richard, and Peto, Richard. *The Causes of Cancer: Quantitative Estimates of the Avoidable Risks of Cancer in the United States Today*. New York: Oxford University Press, 1981.

United States Department of Agriculture. *Ideas for Better Eating*. Washington, D.C.: United States Department of Agriculture, 1981.

United States Department of Agriculture. *Nutritive Value of Foods: Home and Garden Bulletin Number 72*. Washington, D.C.: United States Department of Agriculture, 1981.

United States Department of Agriculture. *Sodium: Think About It*. Washington, D.C.: United States Department of Agriculture, 1982.

Wynder, Ernst L., ed. *The Book of Health*. New York: Franklin Watts, 1981.

Index

233

ABOUT THE AUTHOR

KRISTIN WHITE graduated from Cornell University and began her journalistic career on the *Syracuse Herald Journal*. She has contributed to such diverse magazines as *National Enquirer*, *Cosmopolitan*, *The New York News*, *Free Enterprise* and *Medical World News*. She now specializes in cancer, immunology, virology, molecular genetics, and DNA. She says, "What I know now is the result of the generosity and patience of a number of world-class scientists—Nobel laureates, top-flight researchers, leaders in industry—who've not only educated me, but helped me to make the connection between what I'd learned along the way and what is really new."

She worked on the staff of *Medical Tribune*, and until she left to write this book, she was senior clinical reporter for *Medical World News*. At present she is working on a new book about leukemia, and is a regular contributor to *American Health*, *Medical World News*, *Your Patient and Cancer*, and other magazines for physicians and for the general public.

She lives in New York City and has a grown daughter. Her great joys in life are cooking, traveling, listening to music, and listening to scientists talk about science.

How's Your Health?

Bantam publishes a line of informative books, written by top experts to help you toward a healthier and happier life.

NEED MORE INFORMATION ON YOUR HEALTH AND NUTRITION?

Read the books that will lead you to
a happier and healthier life.

☐ 05024	THE JAMES COCO DIET James Coco & Marion Paone (A Hardcover Book)	$13.95
☐ 23888	ARTHRITIC'S COOKBOOK Dong & Bank	$3.50
☐ 20925	WHAT'S IN WHAT YOU EAT Will Eisner	$3.95
☐ 34106	MY BODY, MY HEALTH Stewart & Hatcher (A Large Format Book)	$11.95
☐ 22872	WOMEN AND THE CRISES IN SEX HORMONES G. Seamans	$4.50
☐ 22673	CONCISE MEDICAL DICTIONARY Laurance Urdange Associates	$4.95
☐ 23335	GH-3-WILL IT KEEP YOU YOUNG LONGER H. Bailey	$3.95
☐ 23827	THE HERB BOOK J. Lust	$4.95
☐ 23767	HOPE AND HELP FOR YOUR NERVES C. Weekes	$3.95
☐ 23818	PEACE FROM NERVOUS SUFFERING C. Weekes	$3.95
☐ 24279	SIMPLE, EFFECTIVE TREATMENT OF AGORAPHOBIA C. Weekes	$3.95

Prices and availability subject to change without notice.